Clinical Applications and Medical Practice

Clinical Applications and Medical Practice

A Guide to Successful Application to Dental and Medical School

First Edition

Vincent S. Gallicchio, Sr.

Clemson University

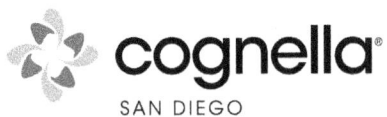

cognella®
SAN DIEGO

Bassim Hamadeh, CEO and Publisher
Craig Lincoln, Project Editor
Samantha Hansen, Production Editor
Emely Villavicencio, Senior Graphic Designer
Laura Duncan, Licensing Coordinator
Natalie Piccotti, Director of Marketing
Kassie Graves, Senior Vice President, Editorial
Alia Bales, Director, Project Editorial and Production

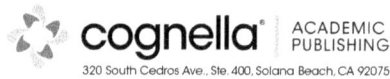

cognella® ACADEMIC PUBLISHING

320 South Cedros Ave., Ste. 400, Solana Beach, CA 92075

Contents

PART I

THE MEDICAL SCHOOL APPLICANT

CHAPTER 1

The Road to Become a Physician/The Road to Medical School

Introduction

Deciding to become a physician has often been considered an admirable career choice. The fact that becoming a physician often leads to a very rewarding career both personally and professionally. Yet, what cannot be ignored is the effort involved to become a physician is both long and often academically arduous. The difficulty involved is centered on the fact that much of the knowledge and skill sets required to become a physician take years to perfect. This means that students of medicine spend many years, at different levels, to master this knowledge. They perfect the specific skills necessary to eventually become a board-certified physician, ready to diagnose and treat patients.

The time involved to become a properly educated and trained physician is a sustained path concentrating on specific focus areas. Within each focus area, there is an expected length of time involved. Within this timeframe is included the comprehension of vast amounts of information and the competency to satisfactorily perform many of the specific clinical procedures. The result intended is that the physician in training becomes artfully skilled and effectively able to eventually treat patients. There is then the requirement to achieve success as demonstrated in each of these focus areas (Patterson et al., 2015; Tartas et al., 2016).

Focus Areas

First Focus Area: Undergraduate Education

The first focus area is the time spent by a student who is interested in becoming a physician, often described as a "premed" student. This first focus area includes the years spent enrolled in a college or university to eventually earn the baccalaureate, that is, BA or BS academic degree. This degree is usually obtained within 4 years. However, during the past several years, undergraduate premed students have been extending the time necessary to graduate (most educational assessments regarding graduation rates include the time taken to graduate within 6 years; Bound et al., 2010). Others will decide to take a "gap year" to improve their overall qualifications, better positioning themselves for successful admission to medical school. The topic of the "gap year" will be discussed in more detail in Chapter 2.

The academic major and the corresponding curriculum chosen by the medical-focused undergraduate student are usually heavily concentrated in the life and/or physical sciences. However, medical schools in general do not specifically recommend any academic major over any other. As long as the interested premedical student becomes knowledgeable, that is, grounded in a general well-rounded liberal arts education that is supported by achieving a significant grade point average (GPA) and by performing as expected on the Medical College Admission Test (MCAT). The emphasis is on the promotion of science, but it is not a detriment to the future medical school applicant to be accepted into medical school if he/she does not select an academic major in a science area. However, they will need to comprehend subjects like biology, chemistry, physics, etc. to perform as expected on the MCAT.

Another topic of increasing importance as part of the undergraduate experience required by medical schools when evaluating applicants for admission is the performance of working, volunteerism, and clinical shadowing. All are performed in a variety of health care facilities such as a clinic, hospital, and private physician's offices (Bound et al., 2010). The importance of clinical shadowing in the medical school admission selection process will be discussed in more detail in Chapter 2.

Assessment of academic performance during an undergraduate period of study is tantamount to determine if the applicant will be successful once enrolled in medical school. Academic performance is determined by gauging the GPA with the vast majority of institutions determining GPA either on a 4.0 or 5.0 scale. The specific GPAs required for medical school acceptance vary with the medical school; suffice to say that the GPA requirement has over the years maintained a steady state. To the contrary, in recent years, the minimum GPA level required to be favorably reviewed by medical school admission committees has increased incrementally (Becker, 2008). In fact, medical school admission committees now require applicants to list separately their overall GPA versus the GPA earned only with the science courses taken (Princeton Review, 2018).

During their undergraduate experience, premedical school applicants are required to take the MCAT. The MCAT can be a deal-breaker for applicants and should be viewed as such by any applicant considering applying to medical school. This topic will be addressed in greater detail in Chapter 2. As stated above, when discussing the importance of the GPA, not all undergraduate baccalaureate degree-granting institutions use the same point system when calculating GPA. Institutions will use either a 4- or 5-point system and when issuing individual letter grades for courses taken, it is not unusual for institutions to offer those letter grades as "+" or "−." This leads to heterogeneity among institutions regarding how they calculate a student's GPA. This creates a dilemma for medical school admission committees—how do they assess the GPA of applicants who attended institutions that calculate their GPA on a 4.0 or 5.0 system with pluses and minuses? The answer is, or to express it in another way, to determine the equalizer among these diverse conditions. That's why all applicants must take the MCAT. The MCAT provides medical school admission committees with the addition information needed to evaluate an applicant's overall academic performance, rather than just their knowledge base when only examining the GPA. The MCAT is the necessary equalizer to offset the GPA when trying to compare academic performance based on different scales (Using MCAT data in 2019 medical school student selection, 2019). It levels the playing field.

Second Focus Area: Graduate/Professional Education

The second focus area is the time spent by the applicant, now as an accepted student in a U.S. medical school accredited by the Liaison Committee on Medical Education (LCME). The 4 years of medical school are focused on overall medical education and learning effective clinical practice. During this time, students will enroll in (on average) 24 academic credits per semester, which is a significant increase compared to their undergraduate academic load. Additionally, laboratory sessions in medical school are much more intense than those taken as an undergraduate (Smith et al., 2016). The accumulated amount of knowledge required for medical students to learn and comprehend over the 4 years of medical school is voluminous.

To address the problem of an ever-increasing amount of knowledge of which students must become proficient, over the past several years medical school curriculum redesign has been initiated. The vast majority of U.S. medical schools are in the process of redesigning their curriculum. For many years the basic medical school curriculum consisted of focusing on the first 2 years, emphasizing the basic sciences. The remaining 3rd and 4th years emphasize the development of clinical skills on how to diagnose illnesses and treat patients afflicted with such illnesses. These are the so called "clinical years." Clinical education during these years takes place at hospitals, clinics, and other health offices located in a variety of geographical areas emphasizing both urban and rural settings.

According to this formula medical students rotate through all general and specific specialties necessary to provide them with a complete view of clinical medical education (Pawlina, 2009). According to the Association of American Medical Colleges (AAMC), such general areas of medical education (years 1 and 2) are clinical medicine, general practice, internal medicine, pediatrics, obstetrics and gynecology, psychiatry, and surgery. Years 3 and 4 are the more specialized areas of clinical medicine such as allergy and immunology, anesthesiology, cardiology, cardiovascular surgery, clinical laboratory sciences, dermatology, dietetics, emergency medicine, endocrinology, family medicine, forensic medicine, gastroenterology, general surgery, geriatrics, hepatology, hospital medicine, infectious disease, intensive care medicine, internal medicine, medical research, nephrology, neurology, neurosurgery, obstetrics and gynecology, oncology, ophthalmology, oral and maxillofacial surgery, orthopedic surgery, otorhinolaryngology, palliative care, pathology, pediatrics, pediatric surgery, physical medicine and rehabilitation, plastic surgery, podiatry, proctology, psychiatry, pulmonology, public health, radiology, rheumatology, surgical oncology, thoracic surgery, transplant surgery, urgent care medicine, urology, and vascular surgery.

With this as a clinical and educational background, especially during the 3rd and 4th year of medical education, students should come to a decision as to what specific area of medical study and specialization they need to select as their professional career choice. With this as a premise, it is in the 4th year of medical education when medical students will then begin the process of applying for their residency program hopefully to receive their top first, second, or third choice. The process of the "match" will be discussed in more detail below and in Chapter 2.

Third Focus Area: Residency

Although they have spent 4 years in medical school, following graduation, graduates are not ready to immediately diagnose or treat patients. There is a need for the next focus area—the medical residency program. As mentioned above, the application for residency begins during the final year of medical school. The process involves what is known as the "Match" (Match a Resident, 2019). The national matching program determines how successful recent MDs are in obtaining their residency program in their specialty of choice. The period of time spent in residency can last anywhere from 3 to 9 years. These "residents" are trained under the supervision of more senior physicians in the medical specialty of choice. The period of time spent in residency is challenging, difficult, and intense with residency usually being the last step in the educational process of clinical training to become a physician, unless one decides to obtain a fellowship for advanced medical clinical training to become an expert.

During residency training, the first year is referred to as the "intern" year (Whitlock, 2019). The difficulty experienced initially by medical graduates to conform to residency, specifically during the intern year, is the amount of work in terms of hours clocked that can add up to as many as 80+ per week. This amount has been reduced from the long-standing practice of interns spending up to or succeeding 120+ hr per week. The amount of work time regarding interns was reduced because of the increased incidence of reported medical mistakes that were attributed to the overworked and sleep-deprived interns, whose collective competencies were compromised due to exhaustion (Baldwin & Daugherty, 2004). Also, regarding the impact of workload on interns during this period, it is often considered part of the workload program to take "call." This is defined as agreeing to work overnight in the hospital setting for up to 36 hr, as part of their 80-hr work week. This is another aspect of the "right of passage." This part of the workload, the taking of call, is typically the requirement of all existing and currently active senior practitioners. It is further expected that all new trainees will have the experience of taking call regardless of the individual's mental or physical state at the time. As mentioned above, the total number of hours a resident may work has been reduced with certain states passing legislation to make this a legal restriction to the total number of work hours a resident may experience in any given week. However, there is more recent commentary that the reduction in the number of hours residents can work has limited their overall competencies in terms of making accurate diagnoses and medical decisions on their patients. This has implications that the maximum work hour rule may shift back to the prior requirement of up to 120 hr per week (Time to lift 16-hr limit on first-year residents, 2019).

Interns may spend an additional 2–4 years beyond their 1st year of residency training fully engaged in medical education and clinical training before they are ready to take specialty board exams to certify their competencies in that medical specialty before being allowed to practice. The overall goal of residency training is to allow the medical graduate to eventually become acutely knowledgeable in that specific field of clinical medicine. During residency training, the resident is subjected to numerous exams and other testing methods to monitor his/her progress toward the goal of being recognized as a medical expert in that specialty.

In 2018, a survey of 75% of medical school deans raised their collective concerns over the growing shortage of medical residency positions. The shortages significantly increase the difficulty medical graduates have in finding a residency of their choice. A shortage of residency positions has contributed directly to current shortages in a variety of medical and surgical specialties, having a distinct impact in meeting the demand for clinical practitioners throughout the country (Factsheet: The resident physician shortage reduction act of 2017, 2018). The AMA in a 2019 study documented that by 2030, there will be an anticipated shortage of 120,000 physicians in the United States (Heiser, 2019; The role of GME funding in addressing physician shortage, 2020). In the 2018 survey, medical school deans also raised concerns over the growing shortages in clinical clerkships and other rotations needed to sustain competencies in clinical medical education. This shortage has been exacerbated by a significant increase in the number of public-financed hospital closures, especially those located in rural communities. Additionally, closures in urban areas and major metropolitan areas across country are also increasing (AAFP, 2016). Collectively, these institutions are referred to often as teaching hospitals. An example is the recent closure of Hahnemann University Hospital in Philadelphia, the major teaching hospital for Drexel University College of Medicine (Rangarajan, 2020). This institution had been responsible for the clinical education of over 570 medical students, residents, and fellows per year. Since 2010, more than 100 rural-based hospitals have closed in the United States with an anticipated 400 more to close in the immediate future (Radcliffe, 2017).

The solution put forth by most health policy and medical education experts in the field is for the federal government to provide more financing in support of overall medical school education and training. However, in the absence of increased federal support, more creative ways to support and underwrite medical education and training are being developed such as cooperative methods to provide the needed finances in the absence of increased federal subsidies (Butkis, 2016). Especially important is to acknowledge that whatever remedy or solution is determined, it must be sustained for a significant number of years (not a band-aid approach needing annual adjustments). The long-term survival of our teaching hospitals and the collective role they play in providing clinical clerkships and residency programs is at stake.

One important distinction from medical education is that medical residents are paid while in a residency program. The hospitals rely on the residents to provide a significant amount of the clinical care needed of patients that enter that hospital, no matter by what means—be it medical emergencies, scheduled surgeries, end stage pregnancy, medical and/or intensive care units, and other means of providing health care to patients.

Upon completion of the residency program, the physician in training takes a final "board" exam. Upon passing the exam that practitioner will refer to him or herself as an expert in that medical specialty and is free to diagnose and treat patients. The newly board-certified physician can apply for positions in various states. Doing so allows them to apply for state licensure granting approval to practice.

Fourth Focus Area: Specific Subspecialty Training

The fourth focus area is the decision by a medical resident in a specific clinical specialty to expand their training to a subspecialty. The goal includes achieving status and recognition as a medical expert and recognized specialist in the field. Such programs are referred to as fellowships (AMA, 2015). Most fellowships last up to 2–3 years and are prominent in areas of medicine and surgery. For example, a surgeon who wishes to focus on pediatrics, specifically dealing with brain cancers among children, may select to engage in a surgical fellowship focused on pediatric neurosurgery.

What Is Allopathic Medicine?

One of the challenges that is not often appreciated by college students needing to understand the process of applying to medical school is that there is more than one path available to achieve the goal of medical school acceptance. Deciding on what path to follow can be a difficult decision, often coupled with confusion about determining "what is the right path for me?" The difficulty is often predicated on a general lack of knowledge regarding which medical school will be the right choice for the applicant (public vs. private; in-state vs. out-of-state) and/or which school will be the best fit based on its curriculum and how this matches the applicant's study habits and career goals.

This dilemma often starts with the premise of not understanding the difference between allopathic and osteopathic medicine. While both produce medical school graduates with similar outcomes, each has their own distinct path of how to achieve this goal. At one time, the two tracks were as far apart as possible in terms of their approach to how best produce medical school graduates. Over time, the differences have now met and often overlap. This development is based upon the identification and better understanding of the similarities that once kept them far apart (Kowarski, 2019). They are becoming blended. Oftentimes, students are not aware that there is even more than one path on this road to medical school acceptance. Let's discuss the similarities and differences between allopathic and osteopathic medicine.

Definition of Allopathic Medicine

Allopathic medicine is sometimes referred to as Western medicine, science-based, or modern medicine. It focuses medical treatment on the use of medicines (pharmaceuticals) and/or surgeries to treat illness. Before the introduction of western medicine, illnesses were treated using a variety of what one would term "home remedies." These included a variety of substances mostly derived from fruits, vegetables, herbs, and other animal and plant products. Each source, depending on how they were processed, produced substances (chemicals) that would contain health-promoting properties. Thus, there is little difference in this approach than what is referred to today as herbal remedies (Herbal Medicine, 2019).

With the advances made in chemical purification and other related process methodologies that became readily available over time, these methods became standard practice. This was first observed about 150 years ago. These advances and standardizations helped launch the beginning of the pharmaceutical industry. Over time, the impetus arose to best understand accurately what substances were present in fruits, vegetables, herbs, or in the animal and plant products that provided relief for the medical condition being studied.

It was generally understood that these naturally occurring compounds ("phytochemicals" meaning they are naturally derived) provide nourishment because they are derived from food. This nutrition is coupled with phytochemicals' propensity to aid in the healing process (Phytochemicals, 2019). Many of these phytochemicals were found to be essential for overall human health. Their absence from the human diet would contribute to the development of a specific disease with a unique pathology. As an example, if a substance such as iron, a trace element, is absent from the human diet, it results in the formation of iron deficiency anemia (Iron and iron deficiency symptoms, 2019). Therefore, a direct correlation exists between the required consumption of a phytochemical via basic human nutrition and the lack of such substance as the causative factor in the development of a human disease. The concept emerged that specific compounds or molecules could be effective treatments for specific human ailments and diseases if applied topically, ingested, or delivered accurately. When such a correlation was established, it demonstrated that these substances could be effective in treating human diseases. They were then referred to as medicines.

The concept of defining naturally occurring molecules as medicine evolved over time. Early researchers went about proving that chemical compounds, once introduced into the human system, could be capable of interacting with a specific physiological process and/or reaction within the body, or effectively inhibit the progress of that process gone wrong. They further affirmed that not using the compounds would lead to a pathological abnormality producing a specific disease of that organ or tissue. It then became apparent that understanding how to employ or use these medicines would be an arduous, complex, expensive, and time-consuming process often requiring years to completely understand the intrinsic nature of these chemical interactions to assist in delaying or reversing a pathological disease process. The advent of using these chemical compounds as "medicine" to prevent, reverse, and/or inhibit a disease process became a skillful art often relying conclusively on science to determine application and efficacy for each human pathological condition the medicine was to be prescribed for clinical use. In contrast, at the same time, there were conditions or circumstances associated with the use of materials advertised as having medical benefits in the absence of sound scientific proof. They were demonstrated to be noneffective for the medical condition, whether generic as in "what ails you" or a specific medical condition (Wachtel-Galor & Benzie, 2011). This created the circumstance of often dealing with the so-called "snake oil salesman."

Chemical compounds were defined as "food," that is, plant and animal products, and it was well understood that they provided active ingredients that at the very least provided proper sustenance of basic nutrition. As a medicine, the chemical compounds rely on their ability to be absorbed through digestion to enter the bloodstream eventually to arrive at the anatomical site where they are best effective in aiding a physiological process or inhibiting a pathological process.

Through the processes of chemistry, it was discovered that molecules acting as single agents, described as drugs, could effectively influence, prevent, and/or treat an ever-increasing list of human diseases. These chemical processes allowed for the extraction, formulation, packaging, and purification of these chemicals (drugs) to be best used as medicines. Combined with the need to best understand the basis of normal physiological systems in non-diseased as well as diseased states, it became well understood that a significant amount of time, effort, and dedication would be required to fully understand these processes. Furthermore, it was important to show how effective such medicines would be when used in the treatment of clinical diseases. A drug's chemistry, pharmacology, and clinical utility in terms of how to best treat patients had to be mastered. The applied use of specific molecules as medicine, both naturally and synthetically manufactured, laid the foundation for the pharmaceutical industry as the entity for this process of drug development to grow.

Understanding how to best medically utilize these drugs serves as the foundation of what has become allopathic medicine. It also refers to the science-based approach using modern methods to treat and prevent human diseases and the necessary time required by physicians to learn how such medicines can be best used as drugs. This has become an essential part of the initial training of physicians in terms of comprehending didactic knowledge to be complemented by clinical training of physicians. Allopathic medicine is then defined as the study of medicine to determine the most effective ways to treat human diseases using conventional methods such as drugs whether they are naturally derived or chemically synthesized.

Currently, there are 155 allopathic medical schools in the United States. Enrollment has increased steadily over the past two decades, on average 43% since 2002. Combined with students enrolled in osteopathic medical schools, the rate over the same period has increased by 63% (Allopathic (MD) medical schools, 2019).

What Is Osteopathic Medicine?

Osteopathic medicine is another branch of human clinical medicine. Individuals who become osteopathic physicians (DOs) attend specific medical schools (referred to as DO schools) for the same period as students attending allopathic medical schools (MD)—4 years (American association of colleges of osteopathic medicine, 2019).

Definition of Osteopathic Medicine

Osteopathic medicine has its origins in 1874 and can be best described as frontier medicine, attributed to the work of Andrew Taylor Still (Osteopathic medicine celebrates 125 years, 2017). The evolution of osteopathic medicine over time was based on the initial rejection of western medicine or pharmaceutical practice as the most effective manner to treat human disease. Its central tenet was to use physical manipulation of bones and joints that allowed the practice to be called "osteopathy" (Doctors of osteopathic medicine, 2019). However, over time the philosophical approach to best treat patients has moved closer to what has been traditionally labeled allopathic medicine. As the two fields have moved closer together in scope and practice, DOs are fully recognized as physicians in all 50 states, 44 international countries as well as an allowed practice to serve in all four branches of the American armed forces (Medical Corps (United States Army), 2012).

There are now 41 DO-accredited schools located in 61 sites in the United States compared to 155 MD-accredited allopathic schools. As of 2018, there are over 145,000 osteopath-trained physicians and osteopathic students in the United States. The greatest number of practicing DOs is in California as compared to North Dakota, Vermont, and Washington, DC, that have the lowest (AAMC Medical Schools, 2018). There has been a 7,891 (2.5%) increase in number D.O. graduates since 2023.

The number of first-year students enrolled in osteopathic medical school has increased steadily from 500 in 1968 to 5,800 in 2008, over 8,400 as of 2019, and 9,575 in 2023 (Student Enrollment-AACOM, 2023). Currently, approximately 11% of all practicing physicians in the United States are DO trained; however, at present more than 25% of all medical students engaged in clinical training are DOs. Therefore, over time, the number of practicing DOs will increase. This is expected to have a positive impact as DOs tend to choose medical specialties that are currently facing workforce shortages such as family medicine, general internal medicine, pediatrics, and primary care (AACOM, 2023).

Significant Differences: Allopathic Versus Osteopathic Medicine

During the latter part of the last century, the training of DOs in the United States has undergone a significant transformation. Most notable during this period has been the standardization that has seen all osteopath medical school graduates perform at least one residency consisting of a year as an intern followed by a minimum of an additional 2 years in residency (Guerra, 2019). The clinical focus during time in osteopathic medical school still centers on the modern use of bone and joint manipulations; however, many are also trained in the use of conventional methods of patient treatment. This can be due in part because of the merger of allowing osteopathic and allopathic medical school graduates to compete for the small number of residency programs (5 W's of the ACGME (MD/DO Merger), 2019). DOs also can be observed effectively treating patients in all clinical areas of human medicine. Thus, in many instances, any significant difference between allopathic compared to osteopathic medicine basically is one of a philosophical difference rather than anything substantive. The continued movement toward overlapping with respect to clinical training with the practice now in place where medical school graduates from either allopathic or osteopathic medical schools compete for the same residency positions only reflects the nature of their similarities versus any concrete differences related to the education of their respective medical students.

Impact of the Flexner Report on Medical Education in the United States

In 1910, the Carnegie Foundation supported the research conducted by Abraham Flexner that was designed to overhaul the practice of medical education at the time. His findings were published in the report entitled "Medical Education in the United States and Canada" (Flexner Report, 1910). Up until the time of the report, the practice of providing medical education was not standardized and at best was not uniformly practiced across existing medical schools. The report provided a first-hand look at the status of medical education in the United States and Canada. The impact of the report totally changed the perspective on how medical schools should function and how best medical students should be educated to become the best-practicing physicians as possible.

Flexner was not a trained physician but was a highly regarded educator at the secondary school level and as a principal. His basic premise was to study the problem as an educator. His report concluded that the best approach in terms of providing a quality medical education to students would require major reforms to the process.

First recommended was the need to focus on the implementation of standards with respect to the overall medical school organization and importantly the curriculum. At the time of Flexner's study, the vast majority of medical schools were operated strictly as for-profit entities and as such the focus was on profit over the quality of the educational product.

Second, schools at the time lacked a concise and/or well-developed apprenticeship program designed to deliver quality education in the clinical setting.

Third, Flexner concluded that most programs lacked institutional goals and objectives with respect to the quality of the education delivered, rather, only concerned for the incentive to generate profit.

Using the German model of medical education practiced at the time, Flexner recommended a complete overall the curriculum. The report emphasized the importance of providing a very strong foundation focused on the basic medical sciences followed by a sustained period of clinical education focused on a "hands-on" approach where patients would actually be physically examined. The impact of the report immediately resulted in the closure of many of the operational schools, especially those that were for profit. Those who decided to remain did so only after adapting the recommendations highlighted in the report. Abraham Flexner was one of the most significant educators of the 20th century and the impact of his contributions to medical education is still in practice today.

What Are AMA/AAMC and AMCAS?

The American Medical Association

The American Medical Association (AMA) is a professional organization that advances the medical profession and promotes the collective interest of licensed and practicing physicians. It emphasizes best practices designed to advance the delivery of health care to patients through public health policies and in the delivery of medical care. Members can be graduates of both allopathic and osteopathic medical schools (https://www.en.m.wilipedia.org/wiki/American_Medical_Association).

The Association of American Medical Colleges

The Association of American Medical Colleges (AAMC) is dedicated to advance the practice of clinical medicine via a focus emphasizing medical education, medical research, patient care, diversity, and inclusion. It provides useful portals on topics of interest to prospective medical students. It provides crucial guidance and information on how to apply to medical school, taking the MCAT and for medical school students needing to acquire information on residency programs and how to apply. It also advocates for greater partnerships between medical school and their respective teaching hospitals to address the ever-increasing focus on delivering quality health care through many challenges such as basic and clinical education and research.

The American Medical College Application Service

The American Medical College Application Service (AMCAS) is the centralized application process required for all interested students considering applying to medical school. The AMCAS is required by the vast majority of those schools. It serves as the prime application process for medical school acceptance. The AMCAS process can be and often is an arduous and time-consuming process not to be neglected by applicants completing their various medical school applications.

What Are AACOM and AACOMCAS?

The American Association of Colleges of Osteopathic Medicine

The American Association of Colleges of Osteopathic Medicine (AACOM) is an organization focused on assisting and maintaining support among schools of osteopathic medicine. It routinely reviews and orchestrates the education and clinical training for students engaged in osteopathic medicine schools across the country. It is representative of administrators, faculty, and students in osteopathic medicine.

The American Association of Colleges of Osteopathic Medicine Application Service

The American Association of Colleges of Osteopathic Medicine Application Service (AACOMAS) is the on-line portal for the centralized application that is used by students interested in applying to osteopathic medical school. It simplifies the process for applicants by providing important information regarding general admission requirements, application instructions, application deadlines by individual schools, and the need to request any waivers.

How Do I Choose My Path? Do I Choose Allopathic or Osteopathic Medicine?

As was mentioned above, a significant number of interested students seeking to embark on a career as a physician are unaware that there are two distinct paths available to them—allopathic and osteopathic medicine. Even if all undergraduate premedical students are aware of these paths, all potential future medical school applicants must understand what actually is meant by allopathic and osteopathic medicine. They must seek information that addresses the differences between allopathic and osteopathic medicine. Albeit these differences are minimal when considering their respective clinical responsibilities in today's health care environment regardless of the path taken, each applicant will eventually achieve their goal to become a clinical practitioner. It is necessary for medical students to determine whether they are best suited to select the allopathic or osteopathic medicine route. They must decide in their own mind if one path best suits them compared to the other.

There are other determining factors involved that will assist the premedical student toward this selection decision. Several have been previously mentioned.

First, in general, the academic requirements set by osteopathic medical schools are less demanding compared to allopathic medical schools. These requirements consist of overall and science GPAs and MCAT scores. Several osteopathic schools have recently made the decision not to require applicants to take the MCAT. This is based on applicant data that suggests MCAT score performance is not a satisfactory determinant to judge how well a student will perform in an osteopathic medical school.

Second, although there is less of a significant difference between the tracks, the opportunity to eventually choose a medical specialty can influence a student's interest in striving for a successful application to either type of medical school. For example, it was once assumed that if a student's goal was to become a physician focused on family medicine or primary care, they were counseled to apply to osteopathic versus allopathic schools. However, if their goal was to become a physician geared to be trained in a medical specialty such as a surgeon or receiving advanced surgical training to become a cardiovascular surgeon, the student would be advised to apply to an allopathic school instead of an osteopathic medical school.

Third, the number of each type of school has increased significantly in the past 10 years. This is due in part to the expanding population, especially among seniors who collectively demand greater access to health care (education). In addition, the retirement of baby boomer physicians will contribute to the country's need to fill the over 120,000 vacancies expected by 2030. As of 2024, there are a total of 196 medical schools in the United States—155 allopathic and 41 osteopathic medical schools. The selection of what type of school over another is and can be an arduous and nerve-raking task.

How Do I Know Which Medical Schools Might Be Right for Me?

As discussed above, selecting a "best-fit" medical school to apply to is a decision that needs to be made after long hours of reading and comprehension of vast amounts of information. Selecting where an applicant should apply is often a very difficult decision to make dependent upon a multitude of determining factors. Adding to this dilemma are the below-mentioned additional factors. Each separately and collectively can complicate the decision-making process by increasing one's stress level. Several of these additional factors are as follows:

Location—where a medical school is located may be an important factor for an applicant to consider. Individuals may be in favor of a rural over urban setting or vice versa. Geographic location should not be overlooked as an important determining factor.

In-State versus Out-of-State—Public versus Private—often best examined together as they can be related based upon several general decisions:

First, all applicants must ask the question—should I apply to an in-state or out-of-state medical school?

Second is the additional issue—should I apply to a public or private medical school? In general—most in-state schools will favor an applicant who has been a permanent resident of that state when compared to an applicant applying as an out-of-state applicant without establishing permanent residency status in the state prior to application. This rule is practiced routinely, especially by public medical schools, but not private medical schools. However, in certain circumstances, if an applicant attends an undergraduate college or university and is considered an out-of-state student, the public medical school in that same state may characterize their view of that applicant as having sufficient "in-state" qualifications. They will view such an applicant as an in-state applicant. For every medical school under consideration, an applicant is best advised to determine before they begin the formal application process—how many in-state versus out-of-state applications are received and what is the percentage of acceptances for each?

Financial Cost—related to both topics mentioned above is the financial cost to attend medical school. According to the AAMC 2023 data, the total average cost to attend a 4-year public medical school is from $218,792 to $268,476 depending on whether you are viewed as an in-state or out-of-state applicant. The total cost to attend a private 4-year medical school is from $223,360 to $363,836. By comparison, it can be considerably less expensive to study medicine at a public medical school than at a private medical school. Notwithstanding in this discussion is whether any applicant applying to either type of medical school would qualify for any type of financial aid and assistance, which is usually contingent based upon the applicant's qualifications such as GPA and MCAT scores. In other words, the higher, the better.

Housing and Living Expenses—as mentioned above regarding the location of the medical school is the cost of housing and living expenses over the 4-year time span of medical school education. Because of the rural medical school location, an applicant may find the cost of housing and living expenses more affordable when comparing the housing and living costs associated with an urban-based medical school.

Curriculum—every medical school applicant should also engage in due diligence regarding evaluating the curriculum of each school. Gauging the teaching philosophy in place at that institution is crucial. Whatever it may be, it should support the goal to educate and clinically train the best group of physicians. The traditional format articulated and implemented as the result of the Flexner Report focuses the attention on the first 2 years of medical school as time to learn the basic medical sciences. This time period is followed by the clinical years of training focused on the 3rd and 4th years of medical school when medical students finally come into contact with patients.

Over the past 10 years, this concept has seen many changes implemented by an increasing list of medical schools. The basic premise for the change is to allow medical students to begin to interact with patients earlier in their medical training. Thus, many schools now allow patient interaction to occur as soon as possible in the curriculum; therefore, any applicant must evaluate what type of program and curriculum appeals to them.

Opportunities, such as Research—other factors to be considered by a medical school applicant in his/her selection process are what other opportunities would I be exposed to if accepted to their institution? Factors that have been stated as important in this area are opportunities to perform research, whether applied, basic, or clinical and whether there are possibilities to become involved in international mission trips offered by an institution. Global Health is a topic of growing interest in most medical schools, both allopathic and osteopathic in the United States.

Should I take a Gap year before applying to medical school? It is an "ah ha" moment when applicants (after 3–4 years of undergraduate study) realize that their qualifications do not meet the required minimum standards deemed necessary by that medical school admission committee to offer an admission. Criteria used by all medical schools both allopathic and osteopathic to review and select those deemed best qualified to earn an admission offer to their school are very difficult and extremely competitive to achieve. The student needs to determine "What do I need to do to e.g., increase my unsatisfactory GPA?" Or "What do I need to do to correct my under performing on the MCAT?" In either or both scenarios, unsatisfactory performance must be rectified to have a medical school application viewed as sufficient to be offered an acceptance.

The student may take time off after graduation before formally applying to medical school. During this "gap" period, the applicant may take additional academic courses (even complete a medicine-related postgraduate degree) to improve their GPA Alternatively, they may use the time to concentrate to optimally perform when retaking their MCAT. Time spent in a gap year can be 1–2. The duration can depend on how successful the student is in raising their GPA and MCAT scores to meet the minimum academic standards required by the medical school. Finally, obtaining a related medical position through employment or volunteerism to prove exceptional performance, demonstrating the ability to excel in the practical aspect of medicine can be achieved. Only then would a prospective applicant be encouraged to reapply.

Summary

The need to attract more exceptional students to consider the medical profession as a viable rewarding and satisfying career is key to sustaining the delivery of high-quality medical care in the United States. The medical field is in the process of determining what can be done to sustain the delivery of quality care in the United States. At the same time, the medical profession is dealing with a shortage of quality trained physicians that if not corrected will increase substantially over the next 30 years. Students who are contemplating pursuing a career in medicine will find the opportunity to become physicians a much less tedious but still challenging process. There has been the addition of a significant number of new medical schools operating in the country now compared to 10 years ago. This creates an opportunity for more students to consider medical school as a viable career choice. Doing so allows the opportunity to correct the current and sustained shortage of quality-trained physicians. The chapter defined many of the current issues pertaining to medical education. It clarified within the medical profession the differences between allopathic and osteopathic medicines. It further introduced the medical school application process.

Weblinks

AACOM	www.aacom.org
AACOMAS	www.aacomas.org
AMCAS	www.amcas.org
AMA	www.ama.org
Flexner Report	www.archive.carnegiefoundation.org/pdfs/elibrary/Carnegie_Foundation.org
LCME	www.lcme.org

References

5 W's of the ACGME (MD/DO Merger). (2019). *Match A Resident.* https://www.blog.matcharesident.com/5-ws-of-the-acgme-merger-mddo-merger/

AAFP. (2016). Growing shortage of clinical training sites challenges medical schools. https://www.aafp.org/news/education-professional-development/20140706preceptstudy.html

AAMC Medical Schools. (2018). Association of medical colleges. https://www.aamc.org/about/medicalschools/

Allopathic (MD) medical schools (2019). https://www.startmedicine.com/app/mdschools.asp

AMA. (2015). Thinking about a fellowship? 5 things to consider. https://www.ama-assn.org/residents-students/residency/thinking-about-fellowship-5-things-consider

AMA. https://www.en.m.wilipedia.org/wiki/American_Medical_Association

American association of Colleges of osteopathic medicine (2019). *AACOM*. https://www.aacom.org/become-a-doctor/u-s-doctor/u-s-colleges-of-osteopathic-medicine

Baldwin, D. C., Daugherty, S. R. (2004). Sleep deprivation and fatigue in residency training: Results of a national survey of first- and second-year residents. *Sleep, 27*(2), 217. https://doi.org/10.1093/sleep/272.217

Becker, C. (2008). Pre-med preparation: The importance of physician shadowing. *Student Doctor Network*. https://www.studentdoctor.net/2008/03/22/pre-med-preparation-the-importance-of-physician-shadowing/

Bound, J., Lovenheim, M. F., Turner, S. (2010). "Why have college completion rates declined? An analysis of changing student preparation and collegiate resources. *American Economic Journal: Applied Economics, 2*(3), 129. https://doi.org/10.1257/app.2.3.129

Butkis, R. (2016). Financing U.S. graduate medical education: A policy position paper of the alliance for academic internal medicine and the American College of Physicians. *Annals of Internal Medicine, 165*(2), 134–1377. https://www.annuals.org/aim/fullarticle/2520466/financing-u-s-graduate-medical-education-policy-position-paper-alliance

Doctors of osteopathic medicine. (2019). https://www.doctorsthatdo.osteopathic.org/?&gclid=Cj0KCQiAgebwBRDnARIsAE3eZjRcvjvNA10Ucwa9KLeFhsl2udpYcgKMaQV-u

Factsheet: The resident physician shortage reduction act of 2017. (2018). https://www.google.com/search?q=reduced+residency+positions&ie=UTF-8&oe=UTF-8&hl=en-us&client=safari

Flexner Report. (1910). Medical education in the United States and Canada: A report to the Carnegie Foundation for the Advancement of Teaching. *The Carnegie Foundation for the Advancement of Teaching*. https://www.archive.carnegiefoundation.org/pdfs/elibrary/Carnegie_Flexner_Report.pdf

Guerra, T. (2019). Can a medical doctor train in an osteopathic residency? *Chron*. http://www.work.chron.com/can-medical-doctor-train-osteopathic-residency-28475.html

Heiser, S. (2019). AAMC. New findings confirm predictions on physician shortage. https://www.aamc.org/news-insights/press-releases/new-findings-confirm-predictions-physician-shortage

Herbal Medicine. (2019). Better Health. https://www.betterhealth.vic.gov.au

Iron and iron deficiency symptoms. (2019). https://www.medicinenet.com/iron_and_iron_deficiency/article.htm

Kowarski, I. (2019). The difference between D.O. and M.D. *U.S News & World Report Education*. https://www.usnews.com/education/best-graduate-schools/top-medical-schools/articles/2019-11-07

Medical Corps (United States Army) (2012). Headquarters, Department of the Army, Military occupational classification and structure. https://www.web.archive.org/web/20120915083410/http://www4.army.mil/FA40/files

Osteopathic medicine celebrates 125 years. (2017). https://www.theo.osteopathic.org/2017/11/osteopathic-medicine-125-years-history

Patterson, F., Knight, A. K., Dowell, J., Nicholas, S., Cousans, F., Cleland, J. (2015). How effective are selection methods in medical education? A systemic review. *Medical Education*, 50, 36. https://doi.org/10.1111/medu. 12817

Pawlina, W. (2009). Basic sciences in medical education: Why? How? When? Where? *Medical Teacher*, 31(9), 787 https://scholar.google.com/scholar?hl=en&as_sdt=0%2C41&as_vis=1&q=aamce+clinical+medical+education&oq=aamc+clinical+medical+ed#d=gs_qabs&u=%23p%3DwqFZFBALLKcJ

Phytochemicals. (2019). Phytochemicals' role in good health. *Today's Dietitian*. https://www.todaysdietitian.com/newsarchives/090313p70.shtml

Princeton Review. Medical school requirements: science GPA, non-science GPA, overall GPA (2018). https://www.princetonreview.com/med-school-advice/gpa-for-medical-school

Radcliffe, S. (2017). Rural hospitals are closing at an alarming rate. *Health News*. https://www.healthline.com/health-news/rural-hospitals-closing

Rangarajan, S (2020). The closure of a historic hospital is an ominous warning sign. *Scientific American*. https://blogs.scientificamerican.com/observations/the-closure-of-a-historic-hosptal-is-an-ominous-warning-sign/

Match a Resident. (2019). Residency program requirements. Lists of IMG friendly residency programs. https:///www.matcharesident.com?gclid=CjwKCAiA3uDwBRBFEiwA1VsajPZySjfKfMEzS8TIN2Z2PUJeWUK5LryxDuNlKHJXbwchSLuoW6XRoCIR0QAvD_BwE

Sindhu, K. (2019). The US is on the verge of a devastating, but avoidable doctor shortage. https://www.qz.com/1676207/the-us-is-on-the-verge-of-a-devasting-doctor-shortage/

Smith, B. R., Kamoun, M., Hickner, J. (2016). Laboratory medicine education at U.S. medical schools: A status report. *Academic Medicine*, 91(1), 107 https://www.ncbi.nlm.nih.gov/pmc/articles/PMC5480607 https://doi.org/10.1097/ACM0000000000000817

Student Enrollment-AACOM. (2019). https://www.aacom.org/reports-programs-initiatives/aacom-reports/student-enrollment

Tartas, M., Walkiewicz, M., Budziński, W., Majkowicz, M., Wójcikiewicz, K., & Zdun-Ryżewska, A. (2016). The coping strategies during medical education predict style of success in medical career: A 10-year longitudinal study. *BMC Medical Education*, 16(186). https://doi.org/10.1186/s12909-016-0706-1

The role of GME funding in addressing physician shortage. (2020). https://www.aamc.org/news-insights/gme

Time to lift 16-hr limit on first-year residents. (2019). *AAFP*. https://www.aafp.org/news/blogs/leadervoices/entry/time_to_lift_16_hour.html

Using MCAT data in 2019 medical school student selection. (2019). https://www.aamc.org/system/files/c/2/462316-mcatguide.pdf

Wachtel-Galor, S., & Benzie, F. F. (2011). Herbal medicine. An introduction to its history, regulation, current trends, and research needs. https://www.ncbi.nih.gov/books/NBK92773

Whitlock, J. (2019). Doctors, residents, and attendings: What's the difference? The doctors on your healthcare team. *VeryWellHealth*. https://www.verywellhealth.com/types-of-doctors-residents-interns-and-fellows-3157293

CHAPTER 2

Review of the Medical School Application Process

Why Is the Selection of an Academic Major, Degree Program, and Undergraduate Curriculum so Important for the Medical School Application Process?

When students decide to attend college, they may make the decision to attend a specific institution based on their immediate and long-term career goals. Obviously, other decisions weigh heavily regarding the college selection of choice such as cost, location and distance from home, and type, such as, should it be a public versus private institution? Addressing career goals for those students wishing to become physicians once the decision has been made regarding selecting the undergraduate institution of choice, brings into focus two important questions—*(1) Once admitted to college, what is the best academic major to select that will best position the student to attend medical school when enrolled along with; (2) What undergraduate degree program, such as, BA or BS best suits the student's health career goal?*

From the perspective of the medical school, they are less interested in what specific academic major a prospective applicant may choose upon selecting their undergraduate degree course of study. What is viewed as most important in any academic decision as it pertains to the curriculum is the inclusion of specific courses that are recommended to be taken because the topics are covered on the Medical College Admission Test (MCAT). Thus, if a student selects an academic major, for example, English, history, or religious studies, it is highly improbable or at best it will be challenging and difficult that the curricula for these majors will allow students to enroll in the science-based courses such as biology, chemistry, biochemistry, physics, and/or psychology/sociology that are topics covered in the MCAT. The academic major requires the student to enroll in specific courses that are required for that major. Students with these majors will need to find alternative ways to supplement their academic experience by enrolling in the science courses that are lacking to best prepare for the MCAT. Students may then be required to have these science-based courses added to their individual curricula perhaps to be taken either during summer school or during a gap year. Therefore, an important question to ask is—*how should a student be advised if their academic major is not a "best fit" with respect to providing the academic background necessary to perform well on the MCAT?* If an applicant does select a "non-science" major, they should put in place an Action Plan on how they will deal with this issue—the lack of a core component of science-based courses in their academic plan of study. As mentioned earlier, these students will find the MCAT a very challenging experience without ways to acquire an understanding of the life and social science material covered in the exam.

What Are the Action Plan Recommendations for Students Who Decide Not to Major in a Concentrated Science Curriculum?

Students deciding not to major in a science-based curriculum would have several options in order to improve their overall scientific knowledge base: several of these options that may be considered are (1) they could select to "minor" in one of the science disciplines, such as, biology, chemistry, etc. This would allow the student to enroll in science-based courses, albeit fewer in number; accumulate fewer total credit hours compared to a major; and allow these courses to be used effectively for the student/applicant to be exposed and to comprehend this important subject information that should allow these premedical applicants to test as best as possible on the MCAT. (2) Students may consider enrolling in science courses during alternative time periods other than the normal academic year (fall and spring semesters).

One such alternative period would be to enroll in these science-focused courses during summer school or at other times that would be convenient and could be available online. This would allow a student to use the "ala-cart" method, meaning they could select specific science-based courses that best suit their individual needs during what should then be a less stressful period compared to their regular fall/spring academic load of coursework. This summer and/or online option would allow them to pace themselves regarding when and how they wish to be exposed to the material and not be pressed or stressed to enroll in such courses during an academic semester when they may already have a full academic load or if a student has decided to graduate early, thus their academic load could be higher in terms of the number of contact hours compared to a student who would rather graduate on time meaning after 4 calendar years. (3) Students may decide to take a "gap year" to enroll in additional courses whether the courses are part of a post-bac, masters' program, or something equivalent. In either case, a post-bac program or masters' program can assist immensely in improving the academic profile of an applicant and their MCAT overall performance by demonstrating to an admissions committee that the applicant can successfully manage and tackle the academic rigor of specialized science-based courses such as biochemistry and/or gross anatomy; or potentially upper-level science courses. And (4) students decide to enroll in an MCAT prep course or utilize other testing methods aid such as online studying using Internet-based tools such as "Ted Talks." Such prep courses have a variety of delivery methods, but they can be costly. Students will need to weigh the benefit of these prep courses in lieu of their cost.

What Is the MCAT?

A successful application to medical school means an applicant has satisfied several major requirements, each with its own degree of complexity and difficulty. It goes without saying that perhaps the most challenging and stressful of these hurdles for applicants to medical school is generating a satisfactory score on the MCAT. The exam was developed and is administered by the Association of American Medical Colleges (AAMC; https://students-residents.aamc.org/applying-medical-school/taking-mcat-exam/). It is recognized as a part of the admission process by most American, Australian, Canadian, and Caribbean medical schools. Implemented in 1926, the exam was always a paper and pencil test up until 2006; however, since 2007 the test is now taken via a computer. The exam is scored per section on a scale of 118–132 with each question worth one point in each of the separate sections: *Biology & Biochemistry, Chemistry & Physics, Critical Analysis & Reasoning Skills; and Psychological & Social Sciences*. Thus, when measuring the cumulative performance outcome, the total score will range from 472 to 528.

The exam test results are valid for a period of 2–3 years depending on the medical school with testing offered 25 times each year starting in January–October during any given admission cycle. With the on-average 1%–2% increase in applicants applying to medical school annually over the past decade, it is then obvious that there has been an increased demand to take the MCAT. With that said, admission committees have thus experienced a steady increase in student applications over the same period. This increase in the applicant pool in any given application cycle will also include applicants who may not have received a medical school acceptance in the prior application cycle, in part, possibly because of poor MCAT performance. Thus, these repeat applicants are now advised to retake the MCAT to increase their score before reapplying. They are recommended also to do so to obtain a more competitive score for that specific medical school where they are keen to receive an acceptance. Thus, each year, admissions committees review resubmitted applications where applicants have now retaken the MCAT, hopefully to have achieved a higher score that would now be reviewed more favorably than the original score taken during their previous application cycle. Because of the increase in reapplications and retake of MCAT, medical schools are now beginning to limit the number of times an applicant may reapply. Three application cycles are now gaining acceptance to be the recommended limit with respect to how many times applicants may reapply to medical school. In this context, taking the MCAT is now limited to a maximum of 5 times.

The MCAT is a standardized, multiple-choice examination developed to assist medical school admissions committees in evaluating an applicant's qualifications for medical school. It allows admission committees the opportunity to evaluate an applicant's problem-solving and critical thinking skills; in addition to understanding basic knowledge in several critical subject areas such as the natural, behavioral, and social sciences. Such courses have been predetermined to be essential to fully comprehend the academic rigors of a medical school curriculum. Consequently, applicants often approach this exam with much trepidation because of the importance to achieve a sufficient score that is deemed satisfactory by an admissions committee.

Medical school admission committees place great weight on MCAT scores as a key indicator in assessing overall potential student achievement in medical school. Importantly, the score also allows committees to compare and evaluate potential academic achievement by applicants when the academic grade point average (GPA) earned at one's undergraduate institution was calculated using an alternative scoring system that can make comparisons difficult. An example is the need to equate the academic GPA earned following the undergraduate experience of one student when based on a 4.0 scale earned at their undergraduate institution when compared to another applicant who earned their GPA, albeit it was based on a 5.0 scale during the time they were enrolled at a different undergraduate institution. How would an admission committee make such a comparison? If student "A" earned a 3.8 GPA at an institution that operated on a 4.0 system, how would the student be compared with student "B" who obtained a 4.8 GPA at another institution that operated on a 5.0 system? Thus, the rationale is that even though applicants may have different GPAs based upon the grading scale used by their respective undergraduate institutions, they each had to take the MCAT. Thus, it serves as the common denominator used by admission committees to adequately compare two applicants with varying scaled GPAs to attain some level of equivalency. This is achieved when all applicants take the same national standardized exam for medical school admission, which is to compare and evaluate their MCAT performance.

Often asked by medical school applicants are the following questions—*How should I approach studying for the MCAT? How much time is necessary? Am I benefited if I take a "course" on how to take the MCAT? Is it worth the cost? What is an acceptable MCAT score? Once taken and a score is attained, is the score sufficient for my application, or should I retake it?*

All the above inquiries are important questions for any applicant. Each question can add to the anxiety and consternation that comes with preparing for and taking the MCAT, in part, because so much is riding on the outcome. Another important fact that is responsible for the level of anxiety and consternation shown among applicants is the exam format. In 2015, the exam was changed significantly, both in terms of (1) the length of time allowed to complete the exam has increased from 5 to 7.5 hr; (2) the addition of 150 questions to the current format compared to the previous test format; and (3) the additional questions are the result of the expansion of subject areas to include psychology and sociology to complement those focused on the life sciences.

Why Was the MCAT Revised?

The major justification for revising the MCAT exam was to account for the significant and ongoing change in population dynamics currently evolving in the United States where the fastest-growing segments of the American population are occurring within the African American and Hispanic populations. During the past several decades, there has been a sustained reduction in the number of minority applicants applying to medical school. This has occurred for several reasons such as, it was recognized that to increase the number of minority applicants to medical school in the present day would require an expanded applicant pool. Having more minorities attend medical school would eventually produce more African American and Hispanic trained physicians. However, along with this rationalization came the notion that it would take at least another generation to allow for the number of minority medical student graduates to become practitioners to reach the percentage of a physician-trained workforce that reflects the increased inclusion of these groups in the American population.

With that as the premise, the AAMC, along with the American Hospital Association, agreed that something needed to be done to ensure that within the current number of medical school graduates, the majority of whom would still be primarily Caucasian, should *at the very least* possess the necessary knowledge and skill sets to understand the psychosocial issues surrounding a changing race and ethnicity patient-based population. At the same time, focusing on improving the number of ethnicity-based practitioners to reflect these changes in population dynamics will take place more slowly; in fact, it may take a generation to overcome.

Impact of the Cost to Attend Medical School

With that said, recently a dramatic change in the paradigm regarding how medical school education will be paid for has taken hold that may alter the educational practice of training physicians in the United States for many years to come. The impetus for this change is centered on determining how medical school education is to be paid for by those accepted, that is, who may or may not be able to know how they will pay for their medical education once they are accepted to medical school. One well-recognized premise was that an ever-increasing percentage of highly motivated and ambitious minority-based academic achievers often decided to choose an alternative health profession other than medicine, in part because the financial impediment to attend medical school is significant. Obtaining a medical education is expensive. For economically challenged students, the cost of medical school was viewed as prohibitive. In addition, to compound the problem, the lack of financial aid to offset the high costs of medical school education for this group was also cited as a serious problem that acted as a disincentive for minority students to apply to medical school. Among these ethnic groups, the high cost of a medical school education remains an issue for potentially all future applicants.

Then in 2018, New York University (NYU) Langone School of Medicine announced that it would provide full tuition for all medical students incoming and currently enrolled. The financial commitment amounted to approximately $55,000 per year per student. The funding assistance provided would cover tuition costs; however, the medical student would still be responsible for their room and board. With that said, health care experts and medical educators have all agreed this free tuition program qualifies as a "game changer," which is an understatement. It is expected that the tuition coverage plan initiated by NYU should be duplicated at other medical schools, and in doing so, it is also expected to collectively allow qualified minority applicants to reconsider medical school as a definite career option. Following the NYU Medical School announcement leading the way to offer free tuition to its medical students, other institutions have since also implemented similar tuition-free medical education. To date, the list includes—the Washington University in St. Louis, the University of Houston, Kaiser Permanente School of Medicine (Pasadena, CA), Weill School of Medicine of Cornell University, Cleveland Clinic Lerner College of Medicine at Case Western University, and the University of Arizona. These institutions will offer free tuition to medical students who agree to pursue careers in primary care medicine.

One would argue that if tuition assistance would be beneficial to the medical student population most in need meaning minority and disadvantaged students, one would ask—what is the position of tuition assistance to those medical schools that operate as historically black colleges and universities (HBCUs)? Former New York City mayor and U.S. Presidential candidate Michael Blomberg recently committed 100 million dollars to HBCU medical schools to support tuition relief (www.abc13.com).

Why Is MCAT so Important for the Medical School Application Process?

As stated previously, the MCAT exam score allows medical school admission committees the opportunity to properly evaluate an applicant's qualifications. In many instances when examining an applicant's qualifications in total, they include (1) successful academic performance as measured by the GPA; (2) a minimum of three to four high-quality letters of reference, two of which most often should be from an academic and one from a health professional, preferred to be a physician; (3) quality time measured in hours spent engaged in clinical shadowing; (4) their MCAT score; and finally (5) what it is referred to as "other stuff." Other stuff is defined as activities performed by applicants that define an admissions committee applicant's true commitment to pursuing medicine as a career. Examples of activities for this category are (a) the opportunity to participate in a medical mission trip, (b) volunteering at a variety of civic/health entities, such as, assisted living facilities, nursing homes, free clinic, hospice care, Meals on Wheels, Habitat for Humanity, Salvation Army, and summer camps; (c) engaging in an activity that either is unique to the applicant and/or reflects the personality of the applicant that would be viewed favorably by a medical school admissions committee. However, when it comes to the overall impact of the MCAT, it is acknowledged that a competitive MCAT score can overcome a subpar GPA performance. This is important because a subpar MCAT score cannot be overcome by a competitive GPA score. This is very important for applicants to understand and how best they can promote their energy to focus on the MCAT as so much resides on achieving an acceptable score.

What Is the Best Recommended Way to Prepare for the MCAT?[1]

The consensus opinion of most physicians, that is, prior MCAT test-takers, there is no best method to prepare for the MCAT. With that said, the "top ten" recommended actions that a premed student should consider to be best prepared to take MCAT are as follows:

1. Take Practice Exams as Often as Possible

This is obvious. MCAT is not an exam tool to test an applicant's memorization capabilities. More importantly, the exam attempts to gage the applicant's capacity to relate scientific knowledge to core scientific theories and principles sometimes referred to as understanding concepts. The other concept tested in the exam is one's ability to assimilate and interpret new information and/or to relate clinical experiences. What is highly recommended to perfect the skills required to master this section of the exam is to practice taking test questions that best match the focus of that section of the exam.

2. Practice, Practice, Practice

The MCAT is an extensive exam in terms of the total number of questions asked, thus the time necessary to complete the exam is arduous—6 hr and 15 min of actual test taking time, in addition to an additional hour dedicated to taking breaks. So, it goes without saying that prior test-taking practice exams are essential, in fact it is obligatory. Practice test taking, to be maximally effective, should be performed under controlled real-test conditions, meaning reproducing the exact environment and test-taking rules is highly recommended.

The purpose of an intense practice philosophy is multifactorial. As a test-taker, knowing the importance of the outcome, that is, test score performance; therefore, mandates applicants engage in sufficient practice testing necessary for the following reasons—it provides a barometer to assess the applicant's knowledge of the subject material and how the applicant is expected to perform when the exam will be taken under controlled testing conditions. Importantly, this time focus allows the applicant to monitor how they would react mentally in real-time to best pace themselves regarding their mental stasis and physical pace of test-taking over the time allotted to complete each section of the exam. It allows the applicant to set the pace required to perform as acutely as possible during all stages of the exam covering the many different sections in terms of overall test material. What also is very important when evaluating the importance of practice tests is practice tests should be taken in their entirety and not in sections or taking breaks during the exam. Breaking up the exam into sections rather than taking practice exams from beginning to end reduces the capacity to be able to address the issue of maintaining stamina over the time given to complete the exam. Pacing is important to maintain the mental and physical stamina required to sustain the many hours of acute mental focus. Thus, the recommendation is to assimilate the real or actual test conditions (1) take as many practice exams as necessary and (2) take the entire exam without any interruptions.

---

1. The commentary is based on a coronavirus pre-COVID-19 scenario. The COVID-19 pandemic caused a significant change in how the MCAT was administered during this period. The overall impact of the COVID-19 on the delivery of academics, MCAT preparation, test taking as well as the overall application process will be focus of a later chapter.

3. Use as Many Educational Testing Supplements as Possible

There are several educational MCAT test-taking aides available for the use by premedical students. They range from online tools such as video clips, tutorials, lectures, and actual classes that are designed as prep aides. Access to these materials ranges from free to an implanting charge (less expensive to expensive depending on the level of support requested). Services that are provided free are the AAMC, Khan Academy, and Ted Talks (https://www.ted.com/talks, https://www.khanacademy.org/coach/dashboard).

4. Use Effective Supportive Material

As stated above, there are several agencies that provide supportive test materials for students to engage in MCAT prep. The Khan Academy provides material that can be helpful, but you need additional MCAT study resources. One of the best test preps is the AAMC, the developer of the exam. You want to obtain as many practice tests as possible and as many practice questions as you can from the AAMC. The questions used in practice tests are derived from old MCAT texts. Thus, the date of old tests will coincide with your actual MCAT than any other test source meaning the sooner old tests are used to obtain test questions, the closer to the time a student takes their specific test. There are now several test prep Apps such as "MCAT," "MCAT Prep," "MCAT Flashcards," "MCAT Question of the Day," "MCAT Innovations," and "MCAT Mastery" are available to download on a number of handheld devices.

5. When Should You Take Your MCAT? When Are You Ready?

Probably the most accurate method to determine if an applicant is ready to take their MCAT exam is best measured by the performance on practice tests. If the score is low (we will discuss the significance of the score below) or if your score does not achieve what you have predetermined is your target score, then you have the best indication necessary to determine whether you are ready to take the MCAT for real. Thus, if your practice scores are not achieving your overall desired test score then you know you are not ready to take the exam for real; therefore, it is highly recommended, *do not take the exam!* Thus, the purpose of practice exam is to gage and determine whether you are ready to take your exam for real, thus it is recommended to take practice tests as many as possible. **If your test scores are not remotely close to your target score, you're not ready to take the exam for real.** One of the biggest mistakes premedical students make is to rush their MCAT preparation studies, thus they take the exam prematurely before they are ready to score at the level that is expected by medical schools. Some students may get lucky in their test performance, but others, and perhaps most test-takers, are not so lucky. If applicants are not ready for the exam, there is nothing wrong with postponing the exam to a later date, thus giving the applicant more time to study and prepare as necessary.

6. Review Science Content and Information Thoroughly

Premedical students regardless of their academic major or degree program of study are required to focus on their academics in general with special attention given to the core science subjects. The objective is for the applicant to apply their knowledge of science to answer the specific questions covered on the MCAT. Applicants must review the overall science content of their course work.

7. Create a Study Plan

The consensus of those prior MCAT takers is that preparation for the test, as stated, is an arduous and time-consuming process. It is then advised to create a study plan. Whether your plan consists of identifying so many hours per day, so many days of the week for how long, that is, weeks and months, the overall time dedicated must be adhered to religiously without exception. With that said, every student is different. A student may decide that their study time is best accomplished when they are alone, if not isolated, while others may decide that a group approach may best serve their study needs. Perhaps this method of study is how the student(s) conducted themselves during their undergraduate studies. The group approach to studying may make the overall experience more enjoyable compared to studying alone, but it may not be the recommended study method for everyone.

8. Maintain a Normal Life as Best as Possible

Whatever an applicant decides will be their plan of study, that is, how many hours per day, how many days per week, how many weeks per month, etc., try to also maintain a normal life cycle as possible. It is essential that as an applicant you maintain proper nutrition and maintain a normal sleep schedule. Any deviation from what may be best described as a normal schedule should be reduced as best as possible. To say the goal is to maintain a normal life schedule as possible also means try to have a balance of non-study activities to help lessen and relieve the stress that is associated with MCAT prep. A balance of study/non-study activities is highly recommended and encouraged to maintain one's mental health status. Try to keep oneself busy with other non-study–related activities. Remember other medical school-related activities are going to be important factors when any applicant is reviewed, thus, if possible, applicants should use their non-MCAT prep time to either conduct research, serve as a volunteer, or engage in additional clinical shadowing experiences while the applicant's MCAT preparation continues. Overall, a blended set of activities will help keep the applicant mentally alert, reduce fatigue, and stay focused all the while improving the medical school application.

9. Pay Attention to Self-Imposed Deadlines Using a Study Schedule

As mentioned earlier, the amount of material covered on an MCAT is extensive and can be daunting to an applicant trying to determine how they will adequately prepare to understand all of the content information included in the various subject areas. Including the practice tests that will be part of any study plan will place great demands on any applicant's time schedule. Distractions are to be avoided as it will be very easy to fall behind in your preparations. Applicants are advised to prepare and use a study schedule as a guide to maintain and stay on time regarding daily activities. Setting a dedicated schedule with appointed deadlines is recommended to be most beneficial.

What Is the Recommended Value of Study Guides or Other Test Preparations?

What about Guides—Does One Work Better Compared to Others?

There are multiple strategies used by students to best study for the MCAT.

1. Kaplan MCAT Complete 7-Book Subject Review

For several years, the most popular study method recommended has been a set of prep books provided by Kaplan basically because it has been the most comprehensive resource available in the market. One reason for the wide recommendation is that it is particularly resourceful for the visual learner as the prep book provides detailed figures, illustrations, and diagrams along with an easy-to-understand and comprehensive explanation of concepts and theories.

The prep books also offer complete and comprehensive subject reviews to aid the medical school applicant to best understand overall theories and concepts. Of real importance as a significant feature is the total number of practice questions available covering all subjects within a typical MCAT. The questions are thorough and comprehensive in scope and detail and importantly, they are about as close as possible to resemble the actual questions given on the exam to the extent of what an applicant can look forward to when they take the real exam. A significant feature designed to improve individual section performance and overall test scores are the quizzes that are listed at the end of each chapter. The purpose of these quizzes is to serve as guide points to allow the student to monitor their progress section by section.

The Kaplan prebooks are well-designed and the language used makes the information given easy to read. A nice added feature within the prep book has margins wide enough to allow the premedical school applicant to make note-taking easier. Another helpful feature that facilitates the learning process is that the book uses what it refers to as the "key concepts" or "bridges" that have been added to strengthen what the premedical school applicants have learned by citing real-world examples of the concept at hand. The explanations for the practice problems are easy to understand and cover sufficient detail.

The practice book has three full-length practice tests available for premedical school applicants. Accordingly, the practice book provides a substantial list of available online resources that allow the premedical school applicant to accompany the text subject material. A unique feature along with the practice book is a pamphlet that can be used very effectively as a review. The pamphlet also contains important equations, formulas, and diagrams all in one location, thus, allowing for that close to the date of the test review of the most important information. It has been a concern that although the practice book is and can be an effective instrument in terms of test preparation, the practice book has been labeled as being expensive. When added to the $315 cost to take the MCAT, it does add to the expense; however, when factoring the overall impact, it can provide the premedical school applicant with respect to optimizing test preparation leading to generating a significant exam score that optimizes one's chance leading to overall medical school acceptance, then the cost is more than justified.

2. Princeton Review MCAT Subject Review Complete Set, 2nd Edition

The review material made available by the Princeton Review consists of seven books that are also highly recommend as a very adequate test guide, in part based on the complexity and depth covering all the various MCAT categories (https://www.princetonreview.com/medical/mcat-test-prep?ExDT=2&gclid

=Cj0KCQjw59n8BRD2ARIsAAmgPmLvoF97py_FYOGOdL02jaojHBjezS1UeY3Eq8Xl6-_5FnAuc2knmloaAk N0EALw_wcB). The Princeton Review provides a very good understanding of the MCAT basics and in addition the Review provides close to 2,400 comprehensive and meaningful practice questions. The Review has been critiqued according to its level of detail, which is exceptional; however, it also has been criticized as being too detailed, thus adding more complexity than is necessary for its purpose. The Review material is presented in a clear and easily understandable format that is complemented with a full assortment of illustrations that are very colorful in their presentation. An important component of the Review is the use of definitions and end of chapter summaries that allow for an easy access that assists in quick identification and location of material to review. The location of the quizzes at the end of each chapter/section allows for an adequate method to gage basic concepts and key facts in each category. To assess one's comprehension of the information, the Review comes with three online full-length practice tests available that have been reviewed as exceptional with a key feature being the practice exams may be more difficult than the actual MCAT.

3. Examkrackers MCAT Complete Study Package, 10th Edition

Examkrackers more often is the recommended MCAT study tool by medical school admissions personnel based on the following—it is a six-book copulation that serves as a complete study guide for MCAT preparation and provides information that is easier to understand by cutting out all the useless fluff. It is packed with useful tips, facts, details, and memorization tools. The questions are also interspersed in a way that is conducive to reinforcement of the information already learned and hopefully understood.

The authors use a plethora of examples to drive both basic and complex concepts in an easy-to-understand format. The explanations provided are usually well-described and detailed. At the end of each text chapter contains test questions that have been described as difficult; they are generally viewed as providing a great opportunity to practice. The books are visual, meaning they contain many useful diagrams and figures that have been critiqued as very effective. However, it has been recommended that you should dedicate sufficient time to this specific study aide because of the complexity and thoroughness of the explanations given; thus, this test aide may not necessarily be the first study aid you should be ready to adjust to the in-depth explanations offered. If applicants start their MCAT preparation and do not have 5–6 months to dedicate to practice, then this text aide might not be the best way to initially practice.

4. The Princeton Review Complete MCAT

This aide book is excellent for candidates who are short on time and need all the exam content covered in a succinct manner. The concept explanations are good and the content review at the end of each chapter leads to ample practice (https://www.princetonreview.com/medical/mcat-test-prep?ExDT=2&gclid= Cj0KCQjw59n8BRD2ARIsAAmgPmLPTA_9PaOPAmtSJUsVGKl1GK_JS1HXTWLgZEWvH2_Kt7LH0ld4Khwa AsiCEALw_wcB).

This aide book also provides online access to four full-length practice tests. This aide book is not as detailed as the other aide books listed earlier, but it serves as a good refresher for the candidates who already have their basics strong and looking for a concise supplementary aide book to give a final touch to a student's test preparation.

5. Sterling MCAT Practice Tests

This aide book covers a couple of subject areas: *Chemical & Physical Foundations and Biological & Biochemical Foundations.* The knowledge required to aide both the sections can be found in this book. It has four practice tests for each subject. This aide book also contains answers and explanations for both the right *and* the wrong answers, which really adds to understanding the logic behind a particular line of questioning. Additionally, it provides online practice tests with diagnostic reports to highlight the strong and weak areas (http://www.kaptest.com/?&mkwid=sxxySVfae_dc&pcrid=338209342222&pmt=e&pkw =kaplan&pgrid=20953693956&ptaid=kwd-12649751&slid=&gclid=CjOKCQjw59n8BRD2ARIsAAmgPmId4c zrHsCv-UtfcaXOPnhfk0s1RqXzVsJqE6seFoT_CXI-vWHH8SoaAn4VEALw_wcB).

6. Kaplan Test Prep MCAT 528: Advanced Prep for Advanced Students

If an applicant has already performed considerable exam preparation and still is looking for additional study material to gain an additional edge, this study aide is recommended. This aide book provides strategies for answering different question types and even dealing with the entire MCAT exam. The aide stresses the skills, techniques, and shortcuts to handle the trickier questions. Moreover, it also provides plenty of practice problems and review videos. This is an excellent educational testing resource (https://magoosh.com/mcat/top-tips-mcat-studying/).

7. Kaplan MCAT Flashcards + App

For people who prefer not to waste lots of time, the Kaplan flashcards are satisfying. The 1,000 odd flashcards contain the key concepts of MCAT in a succinct format that lends itself to a fast and fun learning experience (https://students-residents.aamc.org/applying-medical-school/taking-mcat-exam/).

Future Trends—Will MCAT Become Obsolete?

There is growing commentary that the MCAT should be eliminated. Relying on a single test with the sole purpose to rank medical school applicants according to the science subjects they should have mastered during their undergraduate studies before going to medical school has been questioned. Consequently, the exam has been responsible for a high degree of applicant anxiety and stress, like no other standardized exam taken up to that moment in time as they embark along their long journey to becomes physicians (https://aamc-orange.global.ssl.fastly.net/production/media/filer_public/6b/9b/ 6b9b3807-1ca4-4ed2-a2eb-0c35b0a45f46/essentials_2020_combined_final.pdf).

With that said, during the past several years, there has been a call emanating from a growing number of medical schools to abandon the MCAT and thus remove the burden it places on medical schools to select the best candidates possible knowing that the exam was not always a true indicator predicting an applicant would make a great medical student nor a competent and caring physician. This change in testing seems to be voiced by an ever-increasing number of osteopathic medical schools compared to the allopathic schools, which continue to require applicants to take the MCAT. Time will tell if the allopathic schools have a change in heart to eliminate the need to use the exam as a requirement for admission consideration. It goes without saying that premed students would prefer to have the exam eliminated, while at the time removing a significant source of stress that often complicates the lives of applicants each year.

Another reason to consider reducing the importance of the exam, by whatever means necessary, stems from the issue that there is an insufficient number of medical students representing minority populations currently attending medical school. This situation is troublesome when compared to the number of minority medical students to the current increase in the percent representation of minorities in the make-up of the general population in the country. During the past several decades the percentage of minority populations representative in the country has and will continue to increase. However, the percentage of medical school acceptances of minority applicants has not increased at a comparable level to the rate of growth of these minorities in the general population. This set of circumstances occurs during a physician population in the country that is distant and does not conform to represent the overall population that the medical community serves. What has been the overall core issue is the fact that underrepresented minority student applicants have produced in general lower scores on virtually all standardized tests including the MCAT. The consequences of this testing pattern have been at the core of the decisions made by medical school admission committees to determine who is or is not accepted into medical schools. Relying or placing an extraordinary weight on the outcome of a single exam used as a screening tool to determine who gets into medical schools or not has prohibited far too many aspiring physicians, including many representative minorities, from pursuing their career goals of becoming a physician.

Over time based upon collected data, the reliance on MCAT results to be the major or in some cases the sole determining factor that allows an applicant to be accepted into medical school. Going forward, medical school admissions committees need to ensure that the applicant selection process proceeds keeping in focus diversity, equity, and inclusion. This ensures that disadvantaged minority applicants are given every opportunity to become medical students and eventually physicians who then become more reflective of the percentage of disadvantaged minority groups in the general population in the country.

Consequently, the focus of the current problem is there are many examples where very intelligent, highly motivated students are prohibited from becoming physicians in part because they have a subpar MCAT performance. Therefore, the question is should all applicants dedicate countless hours to best prepare just focusing on their MCAT performance? There are experts who would say that the answer is "no." With that said, how does a medical student applicant spend their time to best prepare the strongest application possible? The interpretation of a score result is important. For example, does a score below 500 mean that the applicant is now not competent to become a physician? The collective response is no, not necessarily. The real indicator is the persistence of the applicant, who demonstrates a sustained positive attitude and the determination necessary for aspiring to become a physician. These qualities appear to be more useful criteria to ultimately determine if an applicant has what it takes to become a competent and capable physician (https://students-residents.aamc.org/applying-medical-school/article/changing-mcat-exam/).

Over time, it has been observed that many of these aspiring applicants who represent underrepresented minorities have often struggled severely with taking standardized tests, and thus underperformed. When evaluating these underserved applicants, it has been shown that many are overwhelmed by the sense of failure when comparing their test performance with that of their peers. This attitude prevails even when the overall performance is viewed as on par with other applicants. When the data was analyzed in 2017–2018, the average MCAT score was 511 out of 528. There are many examples of applicants majoring in rigorous academic disciplines who collectively underperformed on their MCAT, thus prohibiting their further evaluation for medical school acceptance. In this group are applicants who also possess advanced degrees, such as, PhDs. One could argue that they would then be adequately intelligent to successfully compete as an adequate applicant. In many cases, these applicants work tediously to prepare for their MCAT in several different ways, from paying for review courses to perhaps hiring a tutor to assist their preparation. Many spend long days for months on end studying and taking many practice tests often perhaps weekly.

As stated previously, the MCAT assists and simplifies medical school admissions the screening process and is sufficient for predicting student performance on other standardized tests. However, the issue that raises concern is that MCAT performance does not predict overall performance success either in assessing in medical school or in the clinical training that follows. What is much more predictive of future performance as a physician to be predictive of career success are the following: a combination of GPA, personal statement, evaluation of letters of recommendation, and time spent in clinical settings. No one argues against the need for numerous hours and resources to prepare for the MCAT. The question is "Should this be the most important number in the application?" It certainly is now.

The AAMC data from 2017–2019 showed that the admission rate for students with an MCAT score of 501 or less was, on average, only 11% compared to the 56% rate among students with a higher score. A separate AAMC report demonstrated that underrepresented minority students (American Indian or Alaska Native, Black or African American, Hispanic/Latino, Native Hawaiian, or Other Pacific Islander) have a 38% rate of acceptance to medical school compared to the rate of 45% among the well-represented students (Asian and White).

What may serve as examples to justify the change in reliance on the MCAT? The utility of college entrance examinations such as the SAT and ACT is similarly in question, with several colleges and universities considering alternatives. In addition, the College Board now provides an "adversity score." Thus, medical schools could also choose to follow the example of the FlexMed Program now in place at the Icahn School of Medicine at Mount Sinai School of Medicine in New York City, where undergraduate sophomores from any major can apply without the MCAT. An evaluation confirmed that the overall performance of medical students did not differ between FlexMed students and those admitted using traditional criteria.

So why is the MCAT still so important an indicator of predicting medical school performance? In addition to simplifying the admission process, it is a business. As stated, administered by the AAMC, with fees ranging from $315 to $480 for each of the nearly 96,000 applicants who have taken the MCAT over the last 2 years, it is a substantive source of revenue for the AAMC. The AAMC also offers preparation packages such as the Complete Official MCAT Prep Bundle for $268. Other companies such as Kaplan offer preparation courses with costs ranging from $2,500 to $13,500.

While some would argue that the MCAT standardizes curricula across colleges and universities, it does not consider the barriers to students' performance on standardized tests. A low MCAT score does not correlate with poor performance in college. There are many examples where premedical applicants numbering over 10,000 students who applied to medical school within the last 2 years possessing a GPA of 3.60 or higher and MCAT scores 501 or lower are good examples. If the AAMC truly is committed to support a holistic approach when it comes to address the needs of premedical applicants, it should abolish the MCAT and dedicate additional resources to address diversity issues while at the same time identifying admission criteria that strongly correlate with applicants' actual performance in medical school and beyond. Nobody needs the MCAT—not the schools that have plenty of other ways to determine the best candidates and certainly not the students who spend money and devote countless hours preparing for it.

Why Is the Interview an Important Component of the Application Process?

1. "Make or Break" Status

The interview is a very important component of the application process for medical schools. As is often the case, the interview can serve as the very reason why many qualified applicants (on paper) do not receive an acceptance offer to medical school. To put it simply, this is how medical schools generally work their admissions. Medical schools review a tremendous amount of information on every applicant, stated previously as GPA, MCAT, letters of recommendation, personal statements, extracurricular activities, etc., to determine whether an applicant should be invited to an interview at a given medical school. It is a difficult proposition to receive an offer to interview at medical schools, because year after year, medical school admissions committees receive many more applications from qualified applicants than they can ever accept. Therefore, the schools can and are "fussy" following the evaluation. If a premedical applicant receives an interview at a medical school, applicants need to know they are considered "on paper" to be qualified to receive an acceptance. In terms of percentages, it is safe to conclude that any applicant is now more than halfway to getting accepted. Thus, with the number of overall applications and the high quality of those who apply as the standard, it is understandable to reason why medical schools only accept a small percentage of students for the interview process (https://www.prospectivedoctor.com/how-important-is-the-interview-for-medical-school/).

As stated above, any applicant who receives an invitation for an interview is considered qualified to be an acceptable applicant by that particular medical school. At this point in the application process, all applicants are now starting over. The clock is reset. At this stage of the process, the interview performance is generally more important than how the admissions committee has evaluated the applicant when examining the AMCAS application, the so-called "look on paper" evaluation. Thus, it goes without saying that the interview can be a "make-it or break-it" scenario. If an applicant has difficulty expressing themselves in a one-one and a group situation can be detrimental to performing well during the interview, it will be very difficult to get receive an acceptance to medical school regardless of the "paper" stats in terms of superb GPA performance, MCAT scores, or other evaluative measurements used by admissions committees.

The key factor when it comes to the interview is based on the following. Physicians as part of their daily practice often must communicate "bad" or "disappointing" news to their patients. Certain diagnoses have the implication of mortality associated with them. The diagnosis of "cancer" comes to mind, in particular the significance scenario, for example, when the patient is a child. A life-threatening diagnosis can be very traumatic not just for the patient, if old enough to comprehend, but certainly for the parents; therefore, medical schools place great weight on the ability of the applicant to be an effective communicator. If the applicant's only positive attributes are what they have provided in the "paper" requirements but lack the ability to be an effective communicator, admission committees interpret this as a critically important character flaw that selection of such an applicant for medical school has a high degree of probability not to be further considered. This set of characteristics is often reflected in the personality of the applicant and is referred to as the "bedside manner" of a physician. It is essential for medical schools to choose and select applicants who can demonstrate empathy when engaging in their day-to-day duties as a physician.

What Constitutes an Interview?

The actual interview and how it is conducted can be different at each medical school; however, they all have certain components in common; several of which are as follows: (1) there will be one-on-one conversations between a member of the admissions committee and the applicant; (2) there also can be interviews conducted by a team of committee members and the applicant; and (3) there can also be a panel discussion that includes current medical students enrolled at the school and the applicant. Several schools may combine more than one applicant at a time to engage in a panel discussion with members of the admissions committee or an assembled group of student representatives.

Admission committees rely heavily on the opinion of their current students when evaluating applicants. Most often these participating medical students are 4th-year students because they have experienced the current curriculum over their 4 years of study, thus they have an understanding and perhaps an appreciation knowing what qualities are best served in an applicant and future medical student. It could be argued that the time allotted to achieve such an important decision is based on a relatively short conversation. Participating medical students play another important role that is often unrecognized and unappreciated. While the entire interview process and events take place during the day, applicants are "watched" or viewed for any sign of unacceptable or unprofessional behavior of the applicants during their day interviewing. This evaluation takes place also during other interview events such as—on tours of specific facilities and when engaged in a food event such as during a lunch that is often provided by the school during the day and/or any other reception that may take place during the day's activities (https://www.aamc.org/system/files/c/2/356316-shadowingguidelines2013.pdf).

How Does One Prepare for the Interview?

Several recommended tasks are often mentioned as "must do" with respect to performing as constituting the best preparation for the interview. They are as follows:

1. Create a lengthy list of preparation of questions that should be typed as a word document

Then prepare comprehensive and detailed answers for each question. Review them for conciseness and ease of delivery.

2. Have the practice sessions recorded so that they can be analyzed and reviewed

Having the opportunity to view oneself "in action" can be very instrumental in identifying any flaws, especially in the spoken word along with mannerisms that would be viewed as inappropriate or annoying. We often forget or do not even realize how we sound; therefore, having the opportunity to view and listen can be extremely constructive and helpful. A recent example comes to mind. An admissions committee member complained at great length when an applicant, who happened to be female, during an interview struggled consistently pulling on her skirt while she was sitting. Finally, because this activity became so annoying, the committee member said to the applicant "if you were so concerned about the length of your skirt when you were sitting, why did you decide to wear a skirt to begin with?" Something like this that may be initially viewed as insignificant is actually in reality an important factor. Pulling of her skirt according *to that committee member was a big deal* sufficient to completely change the opinion of the committee members' decision to accept the applicant. Thus, what an applicant decides to wear, male or female, can be and is a very important component of the interview, how any member of the committee will react, thus influencing the decision to accept or reject an applicant.

3. Do mock interviews and practice, practice, practice

As the old saying goes "practice, practice, practice …" There is simply no substitute for repeatedly practicing interviewing and doing it in front of a person or persons who know something about the medical interview and those who do not. The physical mannerisms demonstrated by the applicant that can be identified by performing practice sessions, in addition, to evaluating the quality of the responses to specific questions that are routinely asked during a medical school interview, should improve the applicant's performance. In the past several years, several schools have adopted the "MMI" method to perform a portion of the interview. MMI is the ability to place the applicant in a real-case scenario to determine how well an applicant can think on their feet given a specific medical-oriented scenario. Often MMIs are conducted using volunteers as patients who often are experienced in the role-playing for these interviews. Medical schools may often say there is no wrong or correct answer in an MMI, but they are used to gage how well an applicant can "think" on their feet when given a scenario where they have at the most only a few minutes to construct a response. It is conjectured that the MMI process will increase more often as a useful tool that will aid admission committees in making their decisions about who to accept into their medical school.

4. Be cognizant of current topics that may be "in the news" or are popular in opinion

It has been said that medical schools prefer to know that the applicants they are likely to offer an acceptance are individuals who keep abreast of current events, especially those topics that relate to medical or health issues. Such topics are often raised during an interview. To best prepare, it has been advised that applicants should get in the habit of reading the *New York Times* and the *New England Journal of Medicine*. There can be a plethora of topics that are medical or health care in nature that a future physician should know are important for them to gage an opinion. It is not about right or wrong as it is to know a topic is taking the center of attention across the country that may impact their future practice as a physician.

5. Relax and be at ease

During the interview, applicants should try and be as relaxed as possible; however, it goes without saying this may be easier said than done. It is normal to be slightly nervous, but it is more important to try to maintain a sense of normalcy. Applicants do not want to be nervous for the interview, in part, because the outcome of the interview is critical to the acceptance process. A subpar interview can derail the best of applicants no matter what their numbers are on paper or any other achievements they have performed or have accomplished. The interview is very important, and there is something in the adage "first impressions count." An applicant needs to prepare as best they can be due in part because everything mentioned in the AMCAS application is fair game for questioning by an interviewer. Another important ingredient to achieve a successful interview is attitude. If an applicant comes across as being arrogant or cocky, such a determination will derail the best of applicants; therefore, it is the rule of the day for applicants to be humble during the interview process. Arrogance or cockiness will turn off the interviewer. Applicants should view the interview to be a teachable moment and one needs to be willing to both talk and listen.

6. Appearance

As was eluded previously, dressing appropriately can also make or break an interview. For men obtaining a suit is recommended, preferably one that fits well. Shades of blue and gray are most appropriate and preferred. Avoid garish colors and black always since an applicant is not attending a funeral. Thus, having a suit is one of the important things that will dictate the outcome of your interview. It is important to be comfortable, but do not equate comfort with casual. Avoid any desire to wear anything defined as casual attire otherwise the applicant is advised to stay home. Women do not have to wear suits with skirts; however, I remind the reader of the incident stated earlier when addressing what women applicants should wear. It is wise to play it safe and avoid skirts, thus it is appropriate to decide on and select a pantsuit. Shoes also should be selected appropriately, avoid stiletto heels and open-toe shoes. Choose on the side of comfort as the day may require extensive walking that includes going up and down stairs. In summary, wearing the proper attire is incredibly important because interviewers simply will not take an applicant seriously if they are not dressed properly.

7. Read, read, and read more

For any interview, knowledge is a powerful component. It is argued that as an applicant expands their reading, they may not become smarter, but they certainly can become more knowledgeable. Being more knowledgeable lends the applicant to be viewed more favorably and in doing so will allow the applicant to at least appear to be not only more confident but also better prepared to answer any question. When reading what should be read? Recommended readings are books and articles that provide relevant information in a straightforward and efficient manner. There are three major categories worthy for an applicant to focus on *Current events*—Stay in touch with current events, especially politics that may pertain to health care, by viewing/reading articles on CNN, in the *New York Times*, or even Google News. *Medical issues*—Reading about medical topics will probably be the most directly relevant to an applicant's interview process. Read to learn about bioethics, new research and technologies, policies, life as a physician, and medical/scientific thinking. Reading biographies about physicians, aside from spending time with an actual physician, is probably the best and most personal way to learn more about being a physician. As mentioned earlier, having a subscription to the *New England Journal of Medicine* is useful as well because applicants can learn about the latest research, bioethical issues, and policies; and *Personal interests*—Read any books or articles that you as an applicant may find interesting. They can be about anything if the applicant finds joy in reading them. It is not all that inconceivable that it may come to pass that the applicant and interviewer share similar tastes and opinions or have the same favorite book or even movie.

8. What to do after the interview?

Applicants at the end of their actual interview, especially if they have interviewed one-on-one with an interviewer, it is appropriate and recommended to ask for the interviewer's business card and/or contact information. It is advised that applicants should follow up the interview by sending the interviewers a note (usually a handwritten card) thanking them for their time and the opportunity to learn more about their medical school and program. If it is at all possible, when preparing the response, try to remember specific details about the experience and mention these details in your correspondence. For example, if they mentioned that they are doing research in a certain field, you can say something like, "I hope everything goes well with XYZ project."

Another important reason to follow up with an interviewer and to have the interviewer's contact information is to be able to send the interviewer any updates in any category related to your application. The goal to establish a rapport with an interviewer is to have the person serve as a potential advocate for the applicant to the admissions committee. It is acceptable to have the applicant ask the interviewer questions via email, but the correspondence should be kept at a minimum. Finally, it is also recommended following the completion of all the interviews to the schools you were invited to visit, if there is one school that the applicant knows and desires to attend, it is acceptable to forward a letter of intent requesting feedback to inform one specific school that the school is the top choice for medical school. This contact could also be a predicate to highlight and inform the school of any recent significant activities or accomplishments that were not included in the original AMCAS application.

Why Is Clinical Shadowing So Important?

What does it mean to shadow a physician? What should applicants expect from physician shadowing? What is the experience like and what should applicants be looking to gain from it? The overall goal to perform clinical shadowing is to help an applicant confirm that becoming a physician is the correct career choice. One of the best ways to determine what career best suits applicants is to obtain, as best as one can achieve, first-hand exposure to know what it is like to be that specific person who has decided to pursue that specific career. For many career choices, what is required is to participate in an internship. Specifically, for any career in medicine, applicants must attend medical school before they can work as an intern. However, this option is not available to applicants, therefore, the remaining option to understand what it is like to be a physician is the opportunity to shadow physicians. When shadowing physicians, applicants should consider shadowing multiple disciplines, in addition to specific services such as shadowing in the emergency room, surgery suite, night call, and urban and rural clinical settings. This is the only way applicants can assure to appreciate all that is involved when considering becoming a physician noting that the average length of a clinical career can easily last 40+ years, one must be reassured that the profession of choice is then best suited for the applicant. This highlights the importance of the need to shadow physicians as often as possible prior to applying to medical school (https://www.usnews.com/education/best-graduate-schools/top-medical-schools/articles/physician-or-doctor-shadowing-what-medical-school-applicants-should-know).

What Does It Mean to Shadow a Physician?

Shadowing a physician means that an applicant will follow a physician as he or she engages in his or her daily duties. This will include time spent in the office, whether sitting alongside the physician with the time spent in the clinical setting, such as, hospital and/or outpatient clinic. Applicants will observe how the physician interacts with his or her patients, performs procedures, converses with his or her coworkers, and even how he or she spends their time during lunchtime/breaks. It is important to note that the clinical shadowing experience is limited. Health care laws (HIPPA and ACA) prohibit direct contact between a student and patients thus the opportunity is basically one of observation not hands-on experience. Consequently because of the regulations in place, applicants are not expected to do much, but also because their knowledge of medicine is limited. Thus, the clinical shadowing exercise is a truly learning experience.

What Should an Applicant Expect from Physician Shadowing?

There are three parties involved when an applicant shadows: the physician, the patient, and the applicant. There are many benefits to clinical shadowing. The first benefit of clinical shadowing is that it provides the applicant with a great way to build a relationship with the physician. To the applicant, the physician can serve as a mentor, friend, or both. Importantly, the applicant can ask for a letter of recommendation and/or a referral to another physician to shadow. Second, the clinical shadowing experience allows the applicant to engage with directly patients, giving the applicant the opportunity to learn more about specific patients and their ailments. Being present allows the applicant to listen attentively to every patient's story and description why they are seeking medical attention, which can be one of the most important reasons why clinical shadowing can and should be an enjoyable experience. Finally, clinical shadowing of physicians should be a stimulating experience for the applicant. They should come away from each experience with the desire to learn more, in fact, all they can about medicine. Each clinical shadowing experience should be a challenge for applicants. With each clinical shadowing experience going forward, applicants should eventually foresee themselves in the role as a future physician. Thus, clinical shadowing should provide applicants with the opportunity to attain achievable goals to work towards as applicants appreciate and understand what is advised to be their passion to pursue a career in medicine.

What Should an Applicant Expect from the Clinical Experience?

There is an incredible amount of variability in clinical shadowing experience. Depending on the one's schedule, the clinical specialty, the clinical practice setting, the time commitment involved, and importantly the personality of the physician the applicant is scheduled to shadow, the time spent by the applicant to shadow should be an enriching and memorable experience. In other words, the time spent to arrange and perform the clinical shadowing experience should make the effort worthwhile and rewarding. The physician may not involve any applicant directly in any of his/her daily routine, or he/she could be incredibly accommodating and ask the applicant to engage in more ways than the applicant ever thought possible. Often if a rapport can be established between the physician and applicant, it is not unusual for the physician to reach out to extend additional times to repeat the clinical shadowing experience, in addition to providing the opportunity to develop a more personal relationship. No matter how or to what extent the clinical shadowing experience presents itself, when the decision is made to shadow a physician, it is advised to keep all expectations low. As stated previously, all applicants should not be surprised if they are not asked to assist with any procedures or aide in the performance of any medical interviews with patients. As a student, applicants are there primarily as an observer. There are rules and laws in place that regulate what can and cannot be performed; therefore, if the applicant wants the experience to be significant, that applicant must be somewhat proactive and take ownership of the experience.

Why Is It So Difficult to Arrange for Clinical Shadowing?

Arranging clinical shadowing experiences for aspiring premedical students is often a challenge that can frustrate applicants. Often the frustration is the result of a lack of understanding on the part of the premedical student wondering *"why does the practitioner that I have been trying to contact fail to consistently not return my phone calls or answer my emails?"* There are several reasons for this lack of contact: (1) Physicians are very busy engaged in their professional lives, thus for them to take the time to now allow premedical students to shadow them is an additional burden many are not willing to engage; (2) Allowing premedical students to shadow physicians is often viewed simply as "to do so is not in my job-description, nor do I receive any additional compensation for taking the time to have these students shadow"; (3) It is possible the medical institution employing the physician, as a matter of institutional policy simply does not allow their clinical staff to engage in shadowing for a number of reasons, such as liability issues that may come into play by having nonclinical trained personnel side-by-side with physicians and the impact of HIPPA and ACA rules; and (4) The potential that having students physically there when the physician is dealing with his or her patients, could cause the physician to become distracted even for a very short period of time, thus increasing the possibility that the physician may make a medical error that could potentially lead to a medical liability and malpractice case. Overall, the process of learning what it means to become a physician is essential for premedical students when considering a career in medicine. Participation in a variety of clinical activities that provide exposure to diverse health care settings can help achieve this goal for these students. Importantly, these activities often allow pre-medical students to understand and affirm their interest in medicine as a career worthy to pursue.

The premedical student needs to understand that clinical shadowing is different from volunteering. Volunteering provides opportunities for the premedical student that enables the unpaid opportunity to assist and aide in a health care setting. Depending on the clinical environment and the needs expressed by the specific clinic etc., volunteering might include filing paperwork, answering phones, reading a book, or playing a game with a child. *These types of experiences are satisfactory when engaged as a volunteer but are not considered clinical shadowing experiences.* Clinical shadowing experiences are defined when the supervisor in charge is a board-certified physician and not a staff member, which more often can be the situation when the premedical student is in a volunteer situation; therefore, as stated previously, clinical shadowing experiences are observational in nature. The premedical student is observant as the health care professional, such as, the physician provides care to his/her patients. The locations where physicians may engage with the pre-medical student can take place in a variety of clinical settings including hospitals, outpatient clinics, long-term care facilities, and/or private practice. As stated above, it is mandatory that any clinical observation always be conducted under the appropriate supervision of a licensed physician or other licensed health care professional, but preferably a physician.

For the premedical student, the clinical shadowing experience not only provides them the opportunity to introduce the profession of medicine and the day-to-day responsibilities of the practitioner, but importantly, it also offers the physician and/or another practitioner the opportunity to showcase the professionalism, in addition to the ethical practice of their duties and to become culturally sensitive when treating their patients. This addresses the ethical and cultural issues that are in play as addressed before when the ethnicity of the current population of practitioners is Caucasian and when the growing percentage of patients represent other racial groups. Thus, until this racial disparity is reversed, it will remain critical to the clinical shadowing experience for the premedical student to appreciate and understand the cultural awareness and education as the premedical student learns how best to engage with patients with respect to understanding the importance of the patient's rights, privacy, and confidentiality.

Since the primary purpose of clinical shadowing is observation in purpose and scope, the experience should totally focus on the ability of the pre-medical student to examine and watch the physician as he/she performs his or her duties in the clinical setting. It then goes without saying again based on HIPPA and ACA regulations, the premedical student should never engage in any kind of activity that is considered practicing medicine. Examples of these kind of activities include, but are not limited to, diagnosing diseases, such as, administering medications, performing any kind of medical or surgical procedures such as taking blood, suturing, providing medical advice, and/or other tasks generally reserved for the trained health practitioner. The AAMC has advised the following learning objectives that serve as guidelines for the premedical student clinical shadowing experience:

Learning Objectives for the Premedical Student

1. Determine the fit of the profession including aptitude, dedication, and attributes needed to pursue and practice medicine
2. Enhance knowledge of how the patient perspective impacts quality care
3. Better understand the roles of the health care team

Premedical Student Responsibilities

1. Provide proof of required immunizations or immunity (i.e., MMR, Varicella [or had chicken pox], Tetanus, or TB) prior to shadowing
2. Complete HIPAA compliance training or review the training provided by the health care provider prior to shadowing experience
3. Sign an agreement to adhere to a Code of Conduct (institution's)
4. Premedical student should sign an agreement of confidentiality (institution's)

Physician–Premedical Student Agreement

1. Establish how premedical student will be introduced to patients (e.g., "this student aspires to enter medical school")
2. Establish a protocol as to how and when a patient is asked if the premedical student can observe the patient–physician interaction (e.g., informed verbal consent—patient is asked by medical staff during check in; patient's response noted in medical record)
3. Establish boundaries and expectations as to when a premedical student's questions are to be asked and answered (e.g., between patients visits or at the end of a shadowing shift)

How Does an Admission Committee Evaluate Clinical Shadowing?

Performing clinical shadowing is still recognized as an important activity for medical school acceptance, in fact a required expectation by most medical schools when evaluating their applicants. Therefore, medical school admissions committee's will emphasize that their applicants have performed clinical shadowing. With that said there is a growing opinion by several schools, such as, UCLA that performance of clinical shadowing is not a prerequisite for medical school acceptance. This rationale for the change is based on (1) applicants experiencing increasing difficulty in finding acceptable clinical shadowing opportunities, and (2) identification of alternative activities that may substitute for clinical shadowing to gain clinical experience.

For a medical school applicant, the experience of clinical shadowing should be viewed in its totality meaning (1) it allows the applicant to gain factual real-time experience on what it is like to be a physician; (2) it allows the applicant to express the collective set of experiences in other forms of the medical school application such as (a) preparing the Personal Statement and (b) when engaging in the interview. Upon performing clinical shadowing applicants then should be able to verbally express and thoughtfully articulate about their collective set of clinical experiences regarding what they witnessed and also why the clinical shadowing was impactful for them. In either case, written or verbally, applicants are expected to be able to articulate their empathy if they encountered challenging or difficult situations when they are in the presence of patients.

The ability to be proactive in describing what is hopefully a positive set of clinical shadowing experiences as part of the application review process is predicated on a number of factors, such as, (1) not all physicians are approachable when trying to secure a clinical shadowing experience and if they do make themselves available, personality can be a key component of what will hopefully be a positive or negative clinical shadowing experience. There are physicians who engage and enjoy the clinical shadowing experience opportunity that they provide for the cohort of physician "wannabes" and there are those who believe otherwise; therefore the opportunity to articulate a positive experience in or during the interview process will be difficult at best; and (2) physician style may be to move so fast or at such a rapid rate defining their "bedside" method that they can leave an unorthodox impression on the pre-medical applicant to the extent they then find it difficult to understand what the clinical experience was they just experienced. In either case, articulating such a disparity can be challenging in either writing the Personal Statement or Personal Interview. In summary, the quality of the clinical experiences can best serve the applicant in whatever means they will measure by an applicant admissions committee.

Should Premedical School Applicants Perform Research as Undergraduates? Does the Performance of Research Increase an Applicant's Ability to Receive a Medical School Acceptance?

Research in any academic discipline can help someone's med school candidacy, experts say. Conducting research in an academic setting can often improve a medical school applicant's chance of admission; however, the research experience does not automatically lead to acceptance, according to most academic physicians and medical school officials who evaluate applications and overall requirements. The performance of compelling research experience can assist and improve the candidacy of a premedical applicant by complementing their overall qualifications; however, the performance of research cannot compensate for a subpar academic performance, whether is the academic GPA, MCAT performance, or a lack of clinical shadowing experiences.

As a general statement, if an applicant has performed very well academically and has performed as expected on their MCAT, performing research would be recommended to bolster their application; however, if an applicant is viewed as having a subpar academic GPA and/or MCAT score, admissions committees view the time needed to perform and succeed in producing a quality research experience, is not worth it because the time required would be best served to focus on one's academics and MCAT test preparation/performance. To do otherwise is then viewed as being counterproductive and not worth the time. Thus, it will not be viewed as an adequate substitute for academic excellence.

Once the academic requirements have been achieved, medical schools would then recommend premedical applicants devote the time and effort necessary to engage in what still needs to be defined as a positive research experience. There are a cohort of highly motivated applicants who after performing as expected in academic achievement can benefit from engaging in a quality research experience, especially if they desire to apply to a research-intensive medical school. In this scenario, having performed quality research can be a valuable asset to their overall application. Again, no matter what type of medical school is being considered, research performance will not substitute for the expected success in an applicant's academic and MCAT performance.

The only type of research that usually impresses an application committee has been also described as a sincere effort meaning the research was conducted in the context where the applicant obtains an advanced degree, such as, a masters' or doctorate degree and not performed just to amplify the applicant's application. This is not a uniform opinion among medical schools, but it is still a viewpoint in play—commit to research performed for its own sake and not simply to aid the applicant's competitive status. To repeat grades and test scores are typically much more important and evaluative factors in the medical school admissions process than the research experience.

Also, to be considered is the following—there is no expectation that the research even must be medical or even scientific. In other words, it could be a scholarly activity that would encompass, such as, applicants who were English and/or political science majors. Published research articles are not the expectation to gage whether a scholarly activity has been successful. If a premedical applicant has given a presentation about their research, this is considered acceptable. One of the most important factors is that it is essential that the premedical applicants having a research background understand the research project they have participated well enough to be able to explain it, especially during the interview, where the applicant will be asked to describe their work in considerable detail, so they must have a sound understanding of what they have just performed even if they only played a minor role in the project.

It must be said that it is possible to get accepted into medical school without having a research background; however, most medical school applicants do have a research experience to showcase. Understanding research having a solid background in the scientific method is often said is what matters not necessarily the type of research conducted. It is how that research experience fits in context with the rest of that applicant's application that matters, and how it fits in the context of what the applicant had available to them. If an applicant was able to perform an independent project, perhaps who was a science major at a major or research university with a plethora of research opportunities and labs, graduate science programs, and there is an on-campus or an affiliated medical school may be viewed quite differently (possibly less impressively) than that same exact project performed by an applicant who may have attended a liberal arts school in a small town that does not offer any graduate science degree programs and there is no affiliated medical school may be reviewed much more favorably by comparison.

Is There "Other Stuff" That Medical School Applicants Need to Consider When Applying to Medical School?

Helpful information. Medical schools operate on a rolling admissions basis. Not all schools that engage in the application cycle process do this, but most of them do comply; therefore, not every medical school is the same. The rule is the earlier an applicant applies the earlier that the applicant will receive secondary applications. The earlier an applicant gets reviewed then the earlier an applicant will potentially be selected for an interview. The earlier in the application cycle an applicant is selected to have their interview, the earlier the applicant can be reviewed post-interview for an acceptance.

Apply as early as possible in the cycle and provide as much information to have a comprehensive and complete application as soon as possible. An application will not be reviewed until it has been determined by the admissions committee that it is complete. At the same time, avoid the temptation to rush to complete it. In other words, obviously the content that needs to be included is of up most importance. Applicants are reminded that they need to pay attention to every detail but do not sacrifice quality to support an early application. Technically, an applicant must accomplish both—submit a complete application as quickly as possible once the AMCAS portal opens to receive applications, which is June 1st in any given year.

If the premedical applicant knows that the AMCAS application portal opens in May of the year before the applicant hopes to start medical school, then he/she should prepare in advance to generate all the necessary components and have them ready to place in the application. Prepare and plan to have all the parts ready for inclusion. This is essential planning to have the application ready for submission in a timely manner.

What admissions committees are looking for is how well prepared was the applicant for creating and submitting a successful application. If the applicant, for whatever reason, passes the application deadline and is late, this sends a negative message for the admissions committee to consider and that is the applicant is not well prepared. The applicant may also be viewed as disorganized or even worse that the application process itself was not of sufficient priority to ensure that they a full commitment to become a physician and enter health care as a career.

Secondary applications. The same conditions apply with secondary applications. Early completion means early review can lead to early decisions regarding whether an applicant will be asked to interview. Secondary applications all contain tailored questions specific for the medical school, thus the information requested is critically important. Delay returning them in 3–6 weeks after receipt sends a very negative message to admission committee, implying that the applicant is just not interested or disorganized, whether this is true or not. The delay tells the committee that the applicant is just too busy to bother or that they are not really interested in their medical school because perhaps they are working on other secondaries. It is a very negative and telling message.

What Happens When an Admissions Committee Receives an Application? What Is Done with the Data?

Admission committees can manipulate all the data received in an AMCAS application and in doing so, they can manipulate whatever they want with the data. At this stage in the process, the applicant is just a "number" with an aggregate of data, numbers, statistics, personal statement, and reference letters. In reality, an admission committee does not know who an applicant is and they have no idea why the applicant wants to attend their specific medical school.

It is critical for applicants to know—medical schools receive, on average, thousands of applications for their school. Thus, because there are so few available seats at every medical school both for interview slots and final acceptance to fill their limited number of seats, medical schools have to every right to be fussy and choosey on who they accept; therefore, they quickly analyze applications to remove those that will no longer receive additional attention. Thus, it is an effective way to reduce the applicant pile quickly and efficiently. Some medical schools will tell all applicants that they review every application; however, many employ the use what are called "digital measures" to filter and screen applications for key metrics, such as, GPA and MCAT scores to eliminate applications considered "outliers" based on these criteria and metrics. Thus, if an applicant MCAT score and GPA do not meet certain cutoffs based on that specific school, the application is pulled and is shredded. It is no longer considered.

With that said, some medical schools will have processes in place to have a person someone go through what applications are pulled by digital measures that otherwise would be shredded. The goal or objective is to find that one application that seeks to find the one applicant who has shown amazing progress with their GPA; however, maybe they just could not raise their MCAT score high enough to be initially included.

Based upon the metrics identified above, most medical schools are going to filter out the atrocious-looking applications based on this data. They are searching for those applicants who just have not proven themselves academically no matter what other supportive data may include in their application. This data would include all additional clinical shadowing experiences and/or any leadership skills disclosed. Unfortunately, medical schools will still send their secondaries out to those students; however, the goal or objective is to increase the revenue stream by collecting the fees associated with secondary submissions.

As an applicant, the goal is to meet or satisfy the metrics, that is, GPA and MCAT score, to gain further consideration to be interviewed. Once an applicant has proven his/her academic standing, one can feel confident the applicant will receive recognition. This means a person in the admissions office will now scrutinize the application seeking to confirm details of the application, such as, how were individual grade performances? What extracurricular activities were performed? Was research conducted with actual positive measurements? Was a post-bac performed or did they earn a graduate degree? What were the extracurriculars such as hobbies, etc.? Not to be overlooked will be the evaluation of the applicants clinical shadowing and overall related clinical experiences, including medical mission trips. Admission committees are interested in knowing—how many hours total added up were conducted, the variety of the experiences, and if there is anything unusual activity was experienced. Everything the applicant has been exposed to will add to the metrics that will decide whether the applicant is placed in the interview pile versus the rejection pile.

How Important Is the Personal Statement?

Next for evaluation is the Personal Statement. There are straightforward pitfalls with the Personal Statement. For example, if it begins by saying that the applicant has always known they wanted to become a physician and to spend their career in health care, the document will be the reason the application will no longer be considered for further consideration. There is a very high probability that if an applicant stumbles with the Personal Statement there is the likelihood the application will no longer be considered. Simply stated, the admissions committee wants to read why the applicant wants to become a physician, pure and simple. The Personal Statement should reflect the applicant's journey past and going forward.

It has been reported that there are medical schools that do not review Personal Statements because, based on prior experience, they have concluded applicants simply cannot construct an effective Personal Statement, so they are ignored. In these circumstances, admission committees just press ahead to review and make evaluations on the applicant's capabilities using additional criteria, such as additional essays that are required with the secondary applications.

What About Diversity? Should It Be Addressed in the Application?

If the applicant is a member of an underrepresented minority, it behooves the applicant to do their homework to make sure the medical school of interest has an affirmative action program or something equivalent, for example, increased financial assistance such as scholarships and/or reduced tuition. It is important if the applicant can make an addition to the diversity of the class if they were to be considered for admission, thus it behooves the applicant to research the medical school regarding percentage of minority students accepted, etc., to make a decision whether the school is worthy of further consideration.

Are Life Experiences Important and Worth Mentioning?

If there is a life experience that is worthy of mentioning it needs to be communicated. It can make the difference whether the applicant will be considered further. If there is a question about an obstacle that an applicant had to overcome, an admission committee wants to learn that an applicant's life experiences may have been difficult, but the obstacles were overcome. Examples are overcoming the loss of a parent, an illness, and/or economic hardships growing up, etc., are worthy of sharing with an admissions committee.

The Importance of International Health Medical Trip Participation

The necessity for applicants to perform clinical shadowing has generated significant interest in the international health mission trip as an effective instrument to satisfy the requirement to perform clinical shadowing for applicants applying to medical school. At the undergraduate level, based on the formula of the classical study abroad model is a successful method to gain the benefits of an international health mission experience while at the same time earning academic credit.

There are many types of programs available for students to consider. Yes, they come at a cost, but considering their availability, while at the same time with the ability to engage in clinical shadowing at home becoming ever more difficult at best, international programs can be critical to the eventual success of any applicant gaining acceptance to medical school. Programs are available that allow applicants to engage in the health mission experience in many of the underdeveloped countries in the world on all continents, including some of the most resource challenged areas in the world. By engaging in these programs, future medical students can obtain first-hand exposure to observe the health care needs of those most deserving by being on the ground and in doing so can assist in aiding these people (https://islonline.org/about/the-isl-experience/).

The type of activities can vary from performing public health surveys, helping rebuild a dilapidated school, hiking through the jungle to bring medical supplies to a remote village, or perhaps even teaching children fundamental academic and life skills. Programs are often constructed based on the needs of the local communities; therefore, the service aspect of any trip depends largely on which country and program is selected. The takeaways from any mission trip can be life changing whether they may be cultural, educational, health-related, or medical in scope and more impactful than if they were obtained in a classroom.

Are There Risks Not Involved in Participating in an International Mission Trip?

While health care students and licensed providers are often drawn to participate in health mission trips, there are those that believe that these efforts are simply "band-aids" that prevent real resolution of critical health issues in the communities served. In evaluating the merits of these trips when delivered in country, it often is too simplistic an approach to fully understand the importance, the overall intent, and the purpose of the mission trip under consideration. More often these trips are designed to help complement existing in country medical services, often taking place with the assistance and guidance of local medical practitioners. The magnitude of the impact of mission trips may have on underserved populations is the key to any trip achieving success.

Whether the trips are delivered nationally or internationally, there is always something positive to take away from a mission trip; however, it is conceivable that such mission trips could be poorly planned. Thus, proper oversight needs to be performed to best determine what an effective trip versus an imperfect one. Going into a country and doing a few procedures really is only a band-aid; however, that should never be the only interpretation because medical trips are conducted. They are never to be considered as a substitute for the local ability to deliver health care, the problem is usually directed to a lack of resources such as medicines. In that context, such trips can be very effective and thus worthwhile.

Do I Need to Take a "Gap Year"?

During a typical medical school applicant year cycle, students apply to medical school the summer before their senior year; however, students who take a gap year delay the application process to the summer after their senior year, thus giving them time to work on the weakest areas of their medical school application before they apply. What are the benefits to delay the application submission by performing a gap year? Here are several reasons why taking a gap year is deemed important.

1. Improve an applicant's MCAT score
It can be difficult for applicants to prep for the MCAT when they are engaged in a full schedule of academic

classes. Any applicant can then maximize an MCAT score by devoting extra time to prepare for the exam without the additional pressures of school obligations.

2. Complete any missing prerequisites

Postbaccalaureate programs are excellent options for filling required premed courses an applicant might be missing. This is especially pertinent if the applicant was not a science major during their undergraduate studies. A nonscience major as an undergraduate, for example, can satisfy their science requirements on their own time-line free of other extraneous activities.

3. Boost a low GPA with a science-based master's program

If an applicant has a subpar academic GPA that is viewed as noncompetitive for medical school, completion of a science-based master's program can dramatically demonstrate an applicant's competency at the graduate level. You'll want a full year of course work to be completed before any application to medical school is submitted. There are also Special Masters Programs (or SMPs) that are usually affiliated with medical schools that are intended for college graduates who want to enhance their transcript for eventual application to medical school. SMP students often take science courses alongside actual med students.

4. Gain research experience

Based on the information previously discussed regarding the pros and cons of performing research, a full year of working in a research laboratory can be a plus to support a future medical school application. The use of the additional time would be beneficial to have devoted to your primary/secondary applications.

5. Volunteer or work in a medically related field

Many successful medical school applicants have some experience in a hospital, clinic, hospice, or other health care setting. Use the additional time to expand and increase medical shadowing experiences.

6. Take a break from academics

Medical school is an intense, if not rewarding experience. However, before embarking on what will be a strenuous and often mentally and physically demanding experience, use the gap year to recharge an applicant's batteries, as they say, or get an education in the real world. For example, one could work full time, teach, travel, or commit to a personal project that has been ignored.

7. Set up preceptorships with local doctors

We have stated the importance of clinical shadowing, or preceptorships, in the medical school application process. Use the gap year to gain additional experience within the medical profession. Importantly, the additional time can be best served if up until the time one has shadowed physicians in only one kind of specialty, thus the gap year is an opportunity to expand their shadowing experiences in other areas of clinical shadowing.

8. Get better letters of recommendation

It could be possible that the gap year provides an applicant with the opportunity to expand specific experiences that may allow applicants into contact with additional professors, researchers, and physicians who will get to know more effectively applicants and their abilities. Building these kinds of relationships in the field can help you if you are missing an important letter of recommendation.

9. Do more research on potential schools and career paths

Applicants can use the additional time to browse medical school profiles by major, location, concentration more efficiently. Also, the extra time can be used to continue a dialogue with key members of any medical school admissions committee.

10. Reflect on your goals

Use the extra time to determine why does the applicant want to be a physician? If you don't have a good answer, take the time to think about your background and ambitions. Another year in school or a year out in the workforce can help you decide if an MD is right for you.

The Bottom Line: Consistency Is Key

However, if the applicant decides to spend a gap year, it is critical to stay engaged in clinical experiences and community service. Medical schools want to see that an applicant's volunteer efforts extend past the time of an applicant's college graduation.

What Do I Do if I Am Rejected? What Is the Recommended Plan Going Forward?

If any applicant discovers they have received a rejection notice from any of the medical schools that they have applied, although extremely disappointing news, perhaps any applicant can take comfort knowing most applicants who apply to medical school annually are also rejected. On average more than 50,000 students start their medical school careers each year that are derived from the thousands of received applications. In fact, most students who apply to medical school each year are rejected (~60%).

One Common Question Asked by the Rejected Applicant Is, What Will Be the Impact of My Status if I Decide to Reapply?

In general, there are many past and current practicing physicians who fail to have been accepted to medical school the first time they applied. It is not an uncommon circumstance. It is often speculated whether an applicant is at a disadvantage if they reapply compared to the first-year applicant. There are medical schools that prefer to accept the first-year applicant when compared to reevaluating the reapplicant in the next application cycle. If you take two identical applicants, one being a reapplicant, and the other being a first-time applicant, all things being equal, and the first-time applicant has the advantage. The objective of the reapplicant has is the need to explain their application has improved from the application submitted previously. If the reapplication is prepared, it needs to be prepared with the same level of accuracy as the first, but hopefully better.

With that said, it stands to reason, regardless of whether it is an applicant's first, second, or third application, one should not apply to medical school until they are ready to do so. It is counterproductive to rush through an application to meet a predetermined application deadline. In addition to the added cost and perhaps additional work involved, only highlights the need to reapply only when you are ready to do so. If an applicant now must reapply. Here are a few recommended helpful hints that should be attended to as part of the reapplication process.

Step 1. Accurately Reassess Your Medical School Application for the Next Cycle

We all face rejection of one type or another during our lives. How we handle rejection is the key ingredient to maintain one's mental alertness. Once an applicant knows for sure that they have been rejected, there are three ways to proceed: First is to give up entirely, toss in the towel and proceed forward trying to determine the next career option to pursue. Second, upon reapplying, if all that is changed in the reapplication is the date the new application is being created, it literally makes very little sense then to expect to have a different outcome following the submission of the same information as previously submitted. Third, the applicant consciously commits to resubmit by providing brand new application that has been updated.

To go into more detail with each step, the **first step** as a reapplicant is to determine why you weren't accepted during your first medical school application cycle. Accurately assessing the shortcomings of an applicant's application will provide the building blocks from which we'll build an applicant's personalized plan in the subsequent steps.

First, reexamine the application closely and *be honest about its strengths and weaknesses*. Next, reach out to schools applied to and ask if their admissions committee could provide any feedback. Several admission committees will do this, others will not. Applicants can also speak to your premedical advisor as an additional data point, but take their input with a grain of salt, as most premedical advisors are woefully unqualified to provide you with substantiative feedback about getting into medical school. Ideally, applicants want input from those with real admissions committee experience who are invested in applicant success. If applicants don't have a personal contact who may have served on medical school admissions committees, they need to try and seek assistance from other qualified health personnel. An honest and accurate assessment is *critical*. Often, applicants target one aspect as a weakness that is actually fine, often they will overlook a real weakness that played a major role in their rejection.

When identifying a weakness, they are recommended to be stratified in order of significance. If you have an MCAT of 501, make sure your MCAT could be better, but it's not the limiting factor in why you didn't get a medical school acceptance the first time around. If an applicant received three or more interviews and no acceptances, **this is a strong indicator that an applicant's interviewing skills require attention.** Don't forget to consider the less obvious factors affecting an applicant's competitiveness. For example, timing of the application. Even with a rock-solid application, applying late in the process, or waiting longer than the recommended 2 weeks to turn around secondaries can add significant delays to an otherwise strong application. Applicants should also revisit their list of medical schools. Important questions to ask are—Did the applicant apply to enough medical schools? Were they appropriate for the level of competitiveness, or were the applicants applying to too many top tier schools that were out of reach? Did applicants consider DO schools or only MD?

Step 2. Formulate Multiple Reapplicant Plans

Now that a list of the most limiting elements of an applicant's application has been prepared, one should focus to formulate a plan. When formulating a plan, keep in mind there is the AAMC's Holistic Review model, a paradigm designed and developed to assess candidates in the application process. This paradigm is also widely used in some capacity by most medical schools. This admissions process model considers each applicant individually by balancing their academic metrics, such as GPA and MCAT, with their experiences and achievements. The tool is designed to be a more effective way to consider how any applicant may contribute value as a medical student and as a future physician. This is one of the many reasons that emphasizes the importance of a narrative-based application, rather than an application resulting from the commonplace checklist-driven mentality. When an applicant understands what medical schools are concerned about, formulating a plan makes much more sense. Why do medical schools care so much about an applicant's MCAT and GPA? They want to ensure that an applicant can handle the academic rigors of a medical school curriculum and most importantly successfully pass the USMLE Step exams that start with Step 1 after the end of the second year of medical school. Why do medical schools care about an applicant's social skills and ethics? These are the important fundamental components to interacting with patients and being an effective physician that have come to the forefront as highlighted earlier when referencing the disparity between the ethnicity when comparing current physicians with the changing demographics of patient populations. Same with being a team player, or being resilient, as every applicant will inevitably face major and perhaps significant obstacles in each applicant's training career; therefore, consider reapplying as one of the many tests that every applicant's resilience and commitment to medicine. The AAMC has created a list of 15 core competencies that every first-year medical student needs to make sure they understand as they embark on their medical education and training. They are:

Service Orientation

Social Skills

Cultural Competence

Teamwork

Oral Communication

Ethical Responsibility to Self and Others

Reliability and Dependability

Resilience and Adaptability

Capacity for Improvement

Critical Thinking

Quantitative Reasoning

Scientific Inquiry

Written Communication

Living Systems

Human Behavior

The list raises the question—Do medical schools expect all applicants to show competency and/or exposure in any or all these qualities? The consensus is no, but applicants need to be cognizant that they exist and may be used by admission committees in their overall evaluation of applicants. When applicants understand what is lacking or deficient in their application, along with knowing exactly what any medical school is expecting to be included in an application, they should provide the rationale to formulate a comprehensive plan so that it becomes an expected expectation with every applicant. At this stage of plan reevaluation, it can be expected that there will be changes. It's natural to have multiple permutations of any applicant's plan. Depending on the length of the time between applications, it is plausible that an applicant's plan may change during this period. As an example, if a 2-year period is being contemplated between applications, an applicant may decide the time will be best spent focusing more on performing research. While another applicant may decide a different plan may emphasize additional clinical shadowing because the gap period between applications is much shorter, perhaps only a year in duration. Applicants do not need to have what would be described as a prefect plan going forward, it just needs to be the best for the applicant.

Step 3. Strategic Prioritization and Reapplicant Plan Implementation

When multiple medical school reapplication plans have been prepared, the next step in the process is to determine what will be the selection procedure going forward to determine which one is the most desirable for each applicant. Perhaps this is the time for an applicant to revisit the important question as to *why* medical school to endure 4 rigorous years of academic and clinical training in order to become a physician? Reflecting on this important question should provide applicants with insight to prioritize what is most important. At the same time, as an example, if primary care in a rural setting is what an applicant may wish to focus upon, then reapplying earlier in the cycle targeting a medical school that fosters the training of primary care physicians makes all the sense. This reexamination may also put in focus the applicant to consider applying to another allopathic medical school or perhaps applying to an osteopathic medical school may make sense. With that said, if any applicant is laser focused to only consider, for example, a surgical subspecialty or are perhaps even undecided on a medical specialty or subspecialty, perhaps an osteopathic medical school is to be considered. Although there are medical schools in the Caribbean region, the selection of these schools needs to be considered very carefully. They have their limitations, such as, graduates often will have difficulties obtaining a residency position returning to the mainland and they can be very expensive to attend.

At any point in the reapplication process, applicants should consistently evaluate and reevaluate their plans based on the pros and cons of each plan under consideration. At this stage, it is recommended applicants reach out to the admissions committee to engage in a dialogue to prepare the best plan forward that is unique for each applicant.

It goes without saying that many premedical students and now potential applicants often express concerns whether delaying their medical school application a year or two is of any consequence either pro or con. With that said, the basic underlying premise all applicants must comprehend that the road to become a successful physician is not a sprint but an extended marathon, filled with many traps or mine fields. Navigating this path is often the best function of time not speed. Whether or not an extra year is warranted and needed is potentially dependent on several key factors. If an applicant has more to accomplish to prepare the best application as possible; therefore, improve their overall competitiveness, then the additional time is an important strategy to consider.

Step 4. In the Reapplication, What Can Be Recycled and What Must Be New?

In any reexamination of the application is to be considered, every component of the application should be scrutinized very carefully to decide what should stay and what needs to be revised.

Personal Statement

The personal statement is required to be new with every application; therefore, if reapplying the personal statement must be prepared again with a new submission. With that said, when comparing the original essay versus the new one, the new essay may focus on similar themes, but it is advised to update all specifics and other mention of prior experiences that were discussed previously. A good example is as follows, a previous personal statement focused on the concern to help underserved communities and that the applicant expressed how this passion was key to the decision to become a physician. In the new revised personal statement, the applicant can again focus on wanting to help deliver medicine in underserved areas. With the new revised edition, the applicant can add more insightful thoughts to expand the passion and career commitment to pursue medicine.

Letters of Recommendation

Letters of recommendation are more subjective in the assessment made by admission committees when compared to the personal statement. If an applicant is uncertain about the quality and strength of any of letters of recommendation to be submitted on behalf of the applicant, it is recommended the applicant request to have it either removed or replace it with a new letter from another recommender. Knowing what a recommender will say in a reference letter is unknown to the applicant for obvious reasons. Thus, to select someone who can prepare a positive letter is critical. A letter composed that at best speaks in generic terms is basically a negative letter. For example, let's say an applicant requests the instructor of their physics course to prepare a letter; however, it has been 2.5 years since the applicant enrolled in the course and there had been no further contact. Odds are the letter can only speak in general terms with no specific statements addressing the applicant's honesty, integrity, and perhaps no statement whether the reviewer thinks the applicant is worthy to be a medical student, never mind a physician. In this hypothetical case, the applicant is advised to seek a new recommender.

If the applicant has spent time during a gap year engaged in a different, but purposeful activity than when the applicant was an undergraduate student, consider requesting a reference letter from the new supervisor or preceptor. As a general rule, each and every letter composed by all recommenders should be as up to date as possible, thus reflecting the most recent period of time when applicant was under the recommender's supervision.

Employment/Activities Section

If the applicant has performed or has been engaged in any meaningful employment-related activity since the time of the first application, the new information must be updated. However, if there are still employment activities that are still meaningful to the applicant's overall profile, then continuing to list these experiences is still recommended. In any event, when listing employment activities applicants should keep in mind to list the most meaningful and impactful two or three activities.

Step 5. Reconsider a Specific Medical School for Application Consideration

If an applicant is going to go through the trouble to reapply to medical school, the very first matter to contemplate is should the same school or schools be considered for application or should new ones be added to replace those no longer to be considered. This may seem a simple and non-rewarding task; however, to add or sub-track a school can be a deal breaker. This raises the question, should any applicant reapply to the same medical schools in the next application cycle? The correct decision depends on the specific medical school in terms of their policy regarding how they handle the reapplication process. Certain schools have a reapplication policy that expects applicants denied admission to reapply; however, in doing so, usual policy dictates that whatever metric(s) was viewed as being the reason why the applicant was rejected, there is the one hundred percent expectation that those metrics found to be substandard or weak must be corrected, fixed and/or reversed. Otherwise, the applicant is basically wasting their time and money, as well as the time of admissions personnel to again re-read and evaluate an applicant's application. For this reason, medical schools are now placing a restriction on the number of times an applicant can apply to their institutions. This decision is based on data that showed only a certain percentage of reapplicants took the time to address and correct the deficiencies of their application. Thus, admissions personnel viewed the time it took to reevaluate these applications as a waste of valuable time, that is, time best spent to address other important needs; therefore, the limit these medical schools have placed on the number of times an applicant may apply to their school has now been set to three.

Thus, when it comes to reapplying to medical, choose the schools wisely, perhaps selecting quality over quantity, but considering any specific limitations with respect to your individual metrics and the restrictions those schools have in place when it comes to how that school has set their individual metrics for reviewing applicants who are reapplying. Some professionals would advise applicants to apply to too many schools versus applying to too few schools, in order words playing the odds. In the final analysis, how many schools to apply too and which ones will be and should be the discretion of the applicant.

Step 6. Until You Actually Submit Your Reapplication, Refine and Perfect the Plan Forward

Any applicant wishing to achieve perhaps a life-long dream to commit to a career in medicine must start with a successful application to enter medical school. To become a physician relies on a steadfast and persistent quest to achieve the necessary background education and clinical training to become a physician. With that said because of the rigors of the medical school application process mandates perseverance among any applicant to stay the course. The benefits of a successful application to medical school lead to establishing what is hoped to be a successful career as a license physician practitioner.

Summary

A career in medicine as a physician is one of the most rewarding occupations anyone can aspire to become; however, becoming a physician is a long and arduous process taking many years to attain the required education and clinical training. When factoring the number of years starting with 4-years of college followed by 4 years of medical school only allows the medical school graduate to call themselves a physician, but not yet ready to handle the complexities of medicine to treat patients, which require additional years of clinical training first as a resident followed by an internship that can add an additional on average 3 years. Then, if the newly trained physician wishes to further his/her clinical training perhaps in a subspecialty requires the performance of a fellowship that adds another 1–3 years. Thus, the total length of training can amount to (4+4+3+3) or 14 years; therefore, if the premedical student starts their undergraduate education at the age of 18, then by the time they complete their 14 years of clinical training, they can easily be in their early 30s. Quite a timeline for sure. Thus, starting with the application process and all that is involved and required to produce a successful application to medical school requires significant attention to details, compliance with understanding requirements, education to best prepare for entrance exams, focus to complete requirements by deadlines, and persistence to complete the application in a timely manner. This chapter addressed the many components involved in the successful application to medical school followed by a description of the basic and clinical education process every medical student will experience before they graduate followed by the years of clinical training needed in order to become board certified in that specialty and/or subspecialty.

References

www.abc13.com. 09/3/20

https://www.ted.com/talks

https://www.khanacademy.org/coach/dashboard

https://www.princetonreview.com/medical/mcat-test-prep?ExDT=2&gclid=Cj0KCQjw59n8BRD2ARIsAAmgPmLvoF97py_FYOGOdL02jaojHBjezS1UeY3Eq8Xl6-_5FnAuc2knmloaAkN0EALw_wcB

https://www.princetonreview.com/medical/mcat-test-prep?ExDT=2&gclid=Cj0KCQjw59n8BRD2ARIsAAmgPmLPTA_9PaOPAmtSJUsVGKl1GK_JS1HXTWLgZEWvH2_Kt7LH0ld4KhwaAsiCEALw_wcB

http://www.kaptest.com/?&mkwid=sxxySVfae_dc&pcrid=338209342222&pmt=e&pkw=kaplan&pgrid=20953693956&ptaid=kwd-12649751&slid=&gclid=Cj0KCQjw59n8BRD2ARIsAAmgPmId4czrHsCv-UtfcaXOPnhfk0s1RqXzVsJqE6seFoT_CXI-vWHH8SoaAn4VEALw_wcB

https://magoosh.com/mcat/top-tips-mcat-studying/

https://students-residents.aamc.org/applying-medical-school/taking-mcat-exam/

https://aamc-orange.global.ssl.fastly.net/production/media/filer_public/6b/9b/6b9b3807-1ca4-4ed2-a2eb-0c35b0a45f46/essentials_2020_combined_final.pdf

https://students-residents.aamc.org/applying-medical-school/article/changing-mcat-exam/

https://www.prospectivedoctor.com/how-important-is-the-interview-for-medical-school/

https://www.aamc.org/system/files/c/2/356316-shadowingguidelines2013.pdf

https://www.usnews.com/education/best-graduate-schools/top-medical-schools/articles/physician-or-doctor-shadowing-what-medical-school-applicants-should-know

https://islonline.org/about/the-isl-experience/

CHAPTER 3

Residency: Finding a "Match

The Definition of Residency in the Training to Become a Licensed Physician

A *resident physician* is the term used more commonly when referring to a recent medical school graduate serving as a *resident, senior house officer* (in Commonwealth countries), or alternatively, a *senior resident medical officer* or *house officer*. Residents have graduated from an accredited medical school and therefore hold a medical degree, such as, MD, DO, MBBS, or MBChB. Residents, in general, serve or constitute, collectively, the medical *house staff* of a hospital. In other words, they make up the team of caregivers responsible for the care of the in-patients residing in the hospital. The term "resident" refers to the fact that resident physicians traditionally spend most of their training "in house" (i.e., the hospital).

The time spent in residency, or the duration of residencies can range from 3 to 7 years, depending upon the program and specialty. For example, becoming a surgeon requires more time spent in residency compared to becoming a pediatrician. Time spent in residency has evolved into periods of time with definitive descriptions. In the United States, a year in residency begins between late June and early July depending on the individual program. It ends one calendar year later. The first year of residency in the United States is known as an internship, therefore this group of physicians is termed "interns." Depending on the number of years a specialty requires, the term *junior resident* may refer to residents who have not completed half their residency. *Senior residents* are residents in their final year of residency, although this can vary. Some residency programs refer to residents in their final year as *chief residents* (typically in surgical branches). Alternatively, a *chief resident* may describe a resident who has been selected to extend his or her residency by 1 year. In this scenario, a chief resident may have a responsibility to organize the activities and training of the other residents. This scenario is typically the path observed in both internal medicine and pediatrics.

Completing a residency does not always indicate that a physician has completed his or her clinical training. If a physician finishes a residency and decides to further or advance his or her clinical training, this can be accomplished by performing a fellowship. Fellowships are conducted with a focus on the area of medical specialization. In this capacity, he or she is referred to as a "fellow." Physicians who have fully completed their training in a particular specialized field are referred to as attending physicians or consultants (in Commonwealth countries). However, this nomenclature applies only in educational institutes in which the period of training is specified in advance. In privately owned, non-training hospitals, in certain countries, the above terminology may reflect the level of responsibility held by a physician rather than their level of education.

The History of Residency

The history of the creation of the residency as it has come to be known is of interest because it reflects the revolution in medical education and the training of physicians that took place in the latter part of the 19th century. Residency, as an opportunity for advanced training in a medical or surgical specialty, evolved over time from brief and informal programs for additional training in a special area of interest. The first formal residency programs were established in the United States by Sir William Osler (https://en.wikipedia.org/wiki/William_Osler) and William Stewart Halsted (https://en.wikipedia.org/wiki/William_Stewart_Halsted) in Baltimore, MD at the John Hopkins Hospital (https://www.hopkinsmedicine.org/the_johns_hopkins_hospital/). Once these programs of residency training were implemented and recognized for their efficiency and level of practice, the establishment of residency programs became the norm throughout the country. Over time, residency programs became formalized and institutionalized for the principal specialties at the beginning of the 20th century. However, the concept of requiring all medical school graduates to enroll in a residency program was not mandatory. Even in the mid-20th century, residency was not seen as necessary for general medical practice; therefore, only a minority of primary care physicians considered residency training obligatory. However, by the end of the 20th century, at least in the United States and parts of Canada, there were few, if any, first-year physicians who went directly from medical school into independent and unsupervised medical practice. An important factor in this evolution of medical education and clinical training was the result of local, state, regional, and/or provincial governments requiring one or more years of postgraduate clinical training to be mandatory for all physicians to obtain their medical license to practice.

Residency programs are traditionally housed in hospitals or within hospital-based medical systems. This has been the custom since the mid-20th century. The location of these programs combined with the duties and responsibilities of residents would often require residents to live or "reside" in what was then developed—hospital-supplied and/or dedicated housing. Remembering that the overall collective duty of medical residents is to provide quality-based health care for the in-patient population 24 hr a day, 7 days a week, and 365 days a year, the so-called "24/7/365" necessitated the requirement that residents be always available including days, nights, weekends, and holidays. This need created what is generally referred to as "Call," meaning night duty in the hospital. However, for certain programs operating in certain health care systems, Call meant sometimes as frequent as every second or third night for up to 3 years in duration. Often this translated into 180-hr work weeks; however, compensation was minimal, and benefits were usually restricted to room, board, and laundry services. Why was this the accepted norm? Because it was assumed that most young men and women undergoing physician training had few obligations outside of their medical and clinical training at that stage of their careers. Trying to establish and then maintain a normal lifestyle during this period often can be a significant challenge. Especially difficult to maintain during this period of residency would be to sustain a relationship and rear children.

Over time, the first year of practical in-patient care-oriented training following the completion of medical school has long been referred to as the "internship." Even as late as the mid-20th century, most physicians after completing a year of general internship would then enter primary care practice. Following completion of the internship year, residency programs would then be separate from internships, thus allowing internists the opportunity to continue in a residency program located at different hospitals. Thus, only a minority of physicians did full residencies. Now most trained physicians will perform an internship, followed by serving in a residency program to be followed by conducting a fellowship. This will easily take up an additional 5–7 years of training beyond the 4-years of medical school.

In some states of the United States, graduates of approved medical schools may obtain a medical license and practice as a physician without supervision after completing 1 year of postgraduate education (i.e., 1 year of residency; before 1975, and often still, called an "internship"), although most states require completion of longer residencies to obtain a license. Those in residency programs who have medical licenses may practice medicine without supervision ("moonlight") in settings such as urgent care centers and rural hospitals; however, while performing the requirements of their residency, residents are supervised by attending physicians who then must approve of their clinical decisions.

Different specialties differ in the length of training, availability of residencies, and options. Specialist residency programs require participation for completion ranging from 3 years for family medicine to 7 years for neurosurgery. This time does not include any fellowship that may be required to be completed after residency to further subspecialize. In 2015, there were almost 7,000 positions for internal medicine compared to around 400 positions for dermatology. Finally, about options, specialty residency programs can range nationally from over 400 (internal medicine) to just 26 programs for integrated thoracic surgery. Below is a list of medical specialties:

Anesthesiology	Immunology	Pediatrics
Cardiology	Internal Medicine	Physical Medicine & Rehab
Cardiothoracic Surgery	Nephrology	Plastic Surgery
Dermatology	Neurology	Podiatry
Emergency Medicine	Neurosurgery	Psychiatry
Endocrinology	Obstetrics & Gynecology	Pulmonology
Family Medicine	Oncology	Radiology
Gastroenterology	Ophthalmology	Radiation Oncology
General Surgery	Orthopedic Surgery	Regenerative Medicine
Hematology	Otorhinolaryngology	Urology
Hepatology	Pathology	Vascular Surgery

Applying to a Residency Program

Factors That Influence a Residency Application

There are many factors that make an applicant competitive. According to a survey of residency program directors, the following three factors were mentioned by directors over 71% of the time as having the most impact:

Step 1 USMLE score (82%)

Letters of recommendation in specialty (81%)

Personal statement (77%)

Between 50% and 71% also mentioned other factors such as core clerkship grades/Step 2 USMLE score/specialty clerkship grades/allopathic medical school attendance/dean's letter.

These factors often come as a surprise to many students in the preclinical years, who often work very hard to get great grades but do not realize that only 45% of directors cite basic science performance as an important measure. The lack of reliance on grades is a departure from the usual or expected norms by which decisions are made when evaluating applicant performance.

A much more impactful change to the evaluation criteria used to evaluate applicants for residency programs is the change in the grading of the Step 1 USMLE Exam. The scoring of the exam will now be on a Pass/Fail system rather than generating a numerical score. The ramifications this change on the evaluation of applicants for residency are still to be determined. When asked by residency program directors, about the implications of this change on their ability to evaluate qualified applicants, the collective responses were—greater emphasis on Step 2 scores than before, perhaps an enhanced portfolio showing excellence in the performance of research related to the residency program being applied for, and even a reexamination of the MCAT score of the applicant back when applying to medical school.

Electronic Residency Application Service

The Electronic Residency Application Service (ERAS) is the centralized online application service applicants for residency programs will use to submit their application, along with supporting documents to residency programs (https://www.aamc.org/).

The ERAS streamlines the residency application process for applicants, their Designated Dean's Offices, Letter of Recommendation (LoR) authors, and program directors. By providing applicants the ability to build and deliver their application and supporting documents in a timely manner streamlines the process, aiming to make the decision process as effortless as possible. Applying to residency involves a complicated set of steps and decisions. The American Association of Medical Colleges (AAMC) is committed to provide information to help applicants apply smarter for residency (https://www.acgme.org/). The AAMC has curated a series of resources that explain the process and ensure that the residency program to be selected is the right fit for the applicant.

Applicants begin the application process with ERAS (regardless of their matching program) at the beginning of their 4th and final year in medical school. At this point, students choose specific residency programs to apply for that often specify both specialty and hospital system, sometimes even subtracts (e.g., Internal Medicine Residency Categorical Program at Mass General or San Francisco General Primary Care Track). After applicants apply to programs, the programs review applications and invite selected candidates for interviews held between October and February. As of 2016, programs can view applications starting on October 1st.

Interviews

The interview process involves separate interviews at hospitals around the country. Frequently, the individual applicant pays for travel and lodging expenses, but some programs may subsidize applicants' expenses. Generally, an interview begins with a dinner the night before in a relaxed, "meet-and-greet" setting with current residents or staff. Formal interviews with attendings and senior residents are then held the next day, and the applicant tours the program's facilities.

Interview questions are primarily related to the applicant's interest in the program and specialty. The purpose of these tasks is to force an applicant into a pressured setting and less to test his or her specific skills.

To defray the cost of residency interviews, social networking sites have been devised to allow applicants with common interview dates to share travel expenses. Nonetheless, additional loans are often required for "residency and relocation."

International medical students may participate in a residency program within the United States as well but only after completing a program set forth by the Educational Commission for Foreign Medical Graduates (ECFMG) (https://www.aamc.org/). Through its program of certification, the ECFMG assesses the readiness of international medical graduates to enter residency or fellowship programs in the United States that are accredited by the Accreditation Council for Graduate Medical Education (ACGME) (https://www.ecfmg.org). The ECFMG does not have jurisdiction over Canadian MD programs, which the relevant authorities consider to be fully equivalent to U.S. medical schools. In turn, this means that Canadian MD graduates, if they can obtain the required visas (or are already U.S. citizens or permanent residents), can participate in U.S. residency programs on the same footing as U.S. graduates.

The Match

Access to graduate medical training programs such as residencies is a competitive process known as "the Match." After the interview period is over, students submit a "rank-order list" to a centralized matching service. It depends on the residency program they are applying for:

Most specialties—currently the National Resident Matching Program (NRMP) by February

Urology Residency Match Program

SF Match (Ophthalmology/Plastic Surgery)

American Osteopathic Association Match

Similarly, residency programs submit a list of their preferred applicants in rank order to this same service. The process is blinded, so neither the applicant nor program will see each other's list. Aggregate program rankings are tabulated in real time based on applicants' anonymously submitted rank lists.

The two parties' lists are combined by an NRMP computer, which creates stable (a proxy for optimal) matches of residents to programs using an algorithm (https://nam.edu). On the third Friday of March each year ("Match Day"), these results are announced in Match Day ceremonies at the nation's 155 MD and 41 DO programs in the United States. By entering the Match system, applicants are contractually obligated to go to the residency program at the institution to which they were matched. The same applies to the programs; they are obligated to take the applicants who are matched into them.

Match Day

On the Monday of the week that contains the third Friday in March, candidates find out from the NRMP whether (but not where) they matched. If they have matched, they must wait until Match Day, which takes place on that Friday, to find out the specific program and where it is located.

Supplemental Offer and Acceptance Program

Informally called the scramble, the Supplemental Offer and Acceptance Program is a process for applicants who did not secure a position through the Match, with the locations of remaining unfilled residency positions released to unmatched applicants the following day. These applicants are given the opportunity to contact the programs about the open positions. This frantic, loosely structured system forces soon-to-be medical school graduates to choose programs not on their original Match list. In 2012, the NRMP introduced an "organized scramble" system. As part of the transition, Match Day was also moved from the third Thursday in March to the third Friday.

Changing Residency

Inevitably, there will be discrepancies between the preferences of the students and programs. Students may be matched to programs very low on their rank list, especially when the highest priorities consist of competitive specialties like—radiology, neurosurgery, plastic surgery, dermatology, neurology, ophthalmology, orthopedics, otolaryngology, radiation oncology, and urology. It is not unheard of for a student to go even a year or two in a residency and then switch to a new program.

A similar but separate osteopathic match previously existed, announcing its results in February, before the NRMP. However, the osteopathic match is no longer available as the ACGME has now unified into a single matching program. Osteopathic physicians (DOs) may participate in either match, filling either MD positions (traditionally obtained by physicians with the MD degree or international equivalent including the MBBS or MBChB degree accredited by the ACGME, or DO positions accredited by the American Osteopathic Association (AOA).

Military residencies are filled in a similar manner as the NRMP, but at a much earlier date (usually mid-December) to allow for students who did not match to proceed to the civilian system.

The matching process itself has also been scrutinized as limiting the employment rights of medical residents, namely whereupon acceptance of a match, medical residents pursuant to the matching rules, and regulations are required to accept all terms and conditions of employment imposed by the health care facility, institution, or hospital.

The USMLE Step 1 or COMLEX Level 1 score[1] is just one of many factors considered by residency programs in selecting applicants. Although it varies from specialty to specialty, Alpha Omega Alpha

---

1. Scoring has been recently changed to a Pass/Fail system.

membership, clinical clerkship grades, LoRs, class rank, research experience, and school of graduation are all considered when selecting future residents.

History of Long Hours

Medical residency programs traditionally require working schedules that amount to lengthy hours for their trainees. In early times, residents literally resided at the hospitals, often working in unpaid positions during their advanced clinical education. During this time, a resident might always be "on call" or share that duty with just one other practitioner. More recently, a change in residency work schedules has been implemented consisting of 36-hr shifts separated by 12 hr of rest, during 100+ hour weeks.

However, the American public, along with the medical education establishment, recognized that such long hours were counterproductive, since sleep deprivation increases rates of medical errors. This was noted in a landmark study on the effects of sleep deprivation and error rate in an Intensive Care Unit. The ACGME has limited the total amount of workhours to 80 hr weekly (averaged over 4 weeks), overnight call frequency to no more than one overnight every third day, and 10 hours off between shifts (https://www.ecfmg.org). Still, a review committee may grant exceptions for up to 10%, or a maximum of 88 hr, to individual programs. Until early 2017, duty periods for postgraduate year 1 could not exceed 16 hr per day, while postgraduate year 2 residents and those in subsequent years can have up to a maximum of 24 hr of continuous duty. After early 2017, all years of residents may work up to 24-hr shifts. While these limits are voluntary, adherence has been mandated for the purposes of accreditation, though lack of adherence to hour restrictions is not uncommon.

Most recently, the Institute of Medicine (IOM) built upon the recommendations of the ACGME in the December 2008 report *Resident Duty Hours: Enhancing Sleep, Supervision and Safety* (https://nam.edu). While keeping the ACGME's recommendations of an 80-hr workweek averaged over 4 weeks, the IOM report recommends that duty hours should not exceed 16 hr per shift, unless an uninterrupted 5-hr break for sleep is provided within shifts that last up to 30 hr. The report also suggests that residents be given variable off-duty periods between shifts, based on the timing and duration of the shift, to allow residents to catch up on sleep each day and make up for chronic sleep deprivation on days off.

Critics of long residency hours trace the problem to the fact that a resident has no alternatives to positions that are offered, meaning residents must accept all conditions of employment, including very long work hours and that they must also, in many cases, contend with poor supervision. This process, they contend, reduces the competitive pressures on hospitals, resulting in low salaries and long, unsafe work hours.

Supporters of traditional work hours contend that much may be learned in the hospital during the extended time. Some argue that it remains unclear whether patient safety is enhanced or harmed by a reduction in work hours which necessarily leads to more transitions in care. Some of the clinical work traditionally performed by residents has been shifted to other health care workers such as ward clerks, nurses, laboratory personnel, and phlebotomists. It has also resulted in a shift of some resident work toward homework, where residents will complete paperwork and other duties at home to not have to log the hours.

Adoption of Working Time Restrictions

U.S. federal law places no limit on resident work hours. While regulatory and legislative attempts at limiting resident work hours have been proposed, they have yet to be passed. Class action litigation on behalf of the 200,000 medical residents in the United States has been another route taken to resolve the matter.

The American Medical Association (AMA), called for reevaluation of the training process, declaring "We need to take a look again at the issue of why the resident is there (https://students-residents.aamc.org/applying-residencies-eras/applying-residencies-eras)."

On November 1, 2002, an 80-hr work limit went into effect in residencies accredited by the AOA (https://www.ama-assn.org). The decision also mandates interns and residents in AOA-approved programs may not work more than 24 consecutive hours exclusive of morning and noon educational programs. It does allow up to 6 hr for inpatient and outpatient continuity and transfer of care. However, interns and residents may not assume responsibility for a new patient after 24 hr.

The U.S. Occupational Safety and Health Administration (OSHA) rejected a petition filed by the Committee of Interns & Residents/SEIU, a national union of medical residents, the American Medical Student Association, and Public Citizen that sought to restrict medical resident work hours. OSHA instead opted to rely on standards adopted by ACGME, a private trade association that represents and accredits residency programs. On July 1, 2003, the ACGME instituted standards for all accredited residency programs, limiting the workweek to 80 hr a week averaged over a period of 4 weeks. These standards have been voluntarily adopted by residency programs.

Though reaccreditation may be negatively impacted with accreditation suspended or withdrawn for program noncompliance, the number of hours worked by residents still varies widely between specialties and individual programs. Some programs have no self-policing mechanisms in place to prevent 100+ hr workweeks, while others require residents to self-report hours. To effectuate complete, full, and proper compliance with maximum hour work-hour standards, there are proposals to extend U.S. federal whistle-blower protection to medical residents.

Criticisms of limiting the work week include disruptions in continuity of care and limiting training gained through involvement in patient care. Similar concerns have arisen in Europe, where the Working Time Directive limits doctors to 48 hr per week averaged out over a 6-month reference period.

More recently, there has been talk of reducing the work week further to 57 hr. In the specialty of neurosurgery, some authors have suggested that surgical subspecialties may need to leave the ACGME and create their own accreditation process, because a decrease of this magnitude in resident work hours, if implemented, would compromise resident education and ultimately the quality of physicians in practice. In other areas of medical practice, like internal medicine, pediatrics, and radiology, reduced resident duty hours may be not only feasible but also advantageous to trainees because this more closely resembles the practice patterns of these specialties, though it has never been determined that trainees should work fewer hours than graduates.

In 2007, the IOM was commissioned by Congress to study the impact of long hours on medical errors. New ACGME rules went into effect on July 1, 2011, limiting first-year residents to 16-hr shifts (https://nam.edu). The new ACGME rules were criticized in the journal *Nature and Science of Sleep* for failing to fully implement the IOM recommendations.

Research Requirement

The ACGME clearly states the following three points in the Common Program Requirements for Graduate Medical Education:

1. The curriculum must advance residents' knowledge of the basic principles of research, including how research is conducted, evaluated, explained to patients, and applied to patient care.
2. Residents should participate in scholarly activity.
3. The sponsoring institution and program should allocate adequate educational resources to facilitate resident involvement in scholarly activities.

Research remains a nonmandatory part of the curriculum, and many residency programs do not enforce the research commitment of their faculty, leading to a non-Gaussian distribution of the Research Productivity Scale. Meaning the metrics used to evaluate research are not distributed equally for all faculty. In other words, the performance of research by faculty is not a requirement.

Financing Residency Programs

The U.S. Department of Health and Human Services, primarily Medicare, funds the vast majority of residency training in the United States. This tax-based financing covers resident salaries and benefits through payments called Direct Medical Education payments. Medicare also uses taxes for Indirect Medical Education payments, a subsidy paid to teaching hospitals that is tied to admissions of Medicare patients in exchange for training resident physicians in certain selected specialties. Overall funding levels, however, have remained frozen over the last 10 years, creating a bottleneck in the training of new physicians in the United States, according to the AMA (https://www.ama-assn.org). On the other hand, some argue that Medicare subsidies for training residents simply provide surplus revenue for hospitals, which recoup their training costs by paying residents salaries (roughly $45,000 per year) that are far below the residents' market value. Inconsistencies regarding residency staffing are not caused by a Medicare funding cap. Rather by Residency Review Committees (which approve new residencies in each specialty) seek to limit the number of specialists in their field to maintain high incomes. In any case, hospitals trained residents long before Medicare provided additional subsidies for that purpose. Many teaching hospitals fund resident training to increase the supply of residency slots, leading to a modest 4% total growth in slots from 1998 to 2004. However, the total number of available residency positions on an annual basis does not come close to provide for an available position for every graduate of an American medical school in any given year (https://www.cfp.ca/).

Changes in Postgraduate Medical Training

Many changes have occurred in postgraduate medical training in the last 50 years:

1. Nearly all physicians now serve a residency after graduation from medical school. In many states, full licensure for unrestricted practice is not available until graduation from a residency program.

Residency is now considered standard preparation for primary care (what used to be called "general practice").

2. While physicians who graduate from osteopathic medical schools can choose to complete a 1-year rotating clinical internship prior to applying for residency, the internship has been subsumed into residency for MD physicians. Many DO physicians do not undertake the rotating internship since it is now uncommon for any physician to take a year of internship before entering a residency, and the first year of residency training is now considered equivalent to an internship for most legal purposes. Certain specialties, such as ophthalmology, radiology, anesthesiology, and dermatology, still require prospective residents to complete an additional internship year, prior to starting their residency program training.

3. The number of distinct residencies has proliferated, and there are now dozens. For many years, the principal traditional residencies included internal medicine, pediatrics, general surgery, obstetrics and gynecology, neurology, ophthalmology, orthopedics, neurosurgery, otolaryngology, urology, physical medicine and rehabilitation, and psychiatry. Some training once considered part of the internship has also now been moved into the 4th year of medical school (called a sub-internship) with significant basic science education being completed before a student even enters medical school (during their undergraduate education before medical school).

4. Pay has increased. As of May 21, 2021, the average annual pay for a First Year Medical Resident in the United States is $83,737 a year. This works out to be approximately $40.26 an hour. This is the equivalent of $1,610/week or $6,978/month.

5. This pay is considered a "living wage." Unlike most attending physicians (i.e., those who are not residents), they do not take calls from home; they are usually expected to remain in the hospital for the entire shift.

6. Call hours have been greatly restricted. In July 2003, strict rules went into effect for all residency programs in the United States, known to residents as the "work hours rules." Among other things, these rules limited a resident to no more than 80 hr of work in a week (averaged over 4 weeks), no more than 24 hr of clinical duties at a stretch with an additional 6 hr for transferring patient care and educational requirement (with no new patients in the last six) and Call no more often than every third night. In-house call for most residents these days is typically one night in four; surgery and obstetrics residents are more likely to have one in three take Call. A few decades ago, in-house Call every third night or every other night was the standard. While on paper, this has decreased hours, in many programs, there has been no decrease in resident work hours, only a decrease in hours recorded. Even though many sources cite that resident work hours have decreased, residents are commonly encouraged or forced to hide their work hours to appear to comply with the 80-hr limits.

7. For many specialties an increasing proportion of the training time is spent in outpatient clinics rather than on inpatient care. Since in-house Call is usually reduced on these outpatient rotations, this also contributes to the overall decrease in the total number of on-call hours.

8. For all Accreditation Council for Graduate Medical Education (ACGME) accredited programs since 2007, there was a call for adherence to ethical principles (https://www.cmsa.co.za).

Relation to Personal Debt

In a survey of more than 15,000 residents in internal medicine, approximately 19% of residents with more than $200,000 in debt designated their quality of life as bad, compared with approximately 12% of those with no debt. Also, residents with more than $200,000 in loans scored 5 points lower on Internal Medicine in Training Exam than those who were debt-free.

Following a Successful Residency

In Australia and New Zealand, it leads to eligibility for fellowship of the Royal Australasian College of Physicians, the Royal Australasian College of Surgeons, or several similar bodies (https://www.amsa.org/).

In Canada, once medical doctors successfully complete their residency program, they become eligible for certification by the Royal College of Physicians (https://www.nbome.org/assessments/comlex-usa/) and Surgeons of Canada or the College of Family Physicians of Canada (CFPC) if the residency program was in family medicine. Many universities now offer "enhanced skills" certifications in collaboration with the CFPC, allowing family physicians to receive training in various areas such as emergency medicine, palliative care, maternal and child health care, and hospital medicine. Additionally, successful graduates of the family medicine residency program can apply to the "Clinical Scholar Program" to be involved in family medicine research (https://www.massgeneral.org/medicine/internal-medicine/education/residency/categorical).

In Mexico, after finishing their residency, physicians obtain the degree of "Specialist," which renders them eligible for certification and fellowship, depending on the field of practice.

In South Africa, successful completion of residency leads to board certification as a specialist with the Health Professions Council and eligibility for the fellowship of the Colleges of Medicine of South Africa (https://www.cmsa.co.za).

In the United States, it leads to eligibility for board certification and membership/fellowship in several specialty colleges and academies.

The Future is Here—Combined Allopathic and Osteopathic Path to Residency

Significant changes to medical education always take time to roll out. The gap between an official announcement and the date when a new process or system begins is often so long that it can easily sneak up on you. Look no further than the DO–MD merger, which combines the allopathic and osteopathic graduate medical education accreditation systems, for proof (https://www.nrmp.org).

The ACGME, the AOA, and the American Association of Colleges of Osteopathic Medicine announced an agreement to move toward a single system for accrediting residency programs back in 2014 (https://www.citizen.org). But the change officially took place on July 1, 2020. Residencies will no longer be MD or DO—they'll all be grouped together (https://www.royalcollege.ca/rcsite/home-e).

Now that the transition to the single system has been initiated, current and soon-to-be medical students have started to take notice. What does the DO–MD merger mean for the future? Will applicants face new obstacles or advantages? The good news is that moving to one system is a lot less scary than it sounds. Here's a breakdown of what every medical student should know about the future of residency training (Supplemental Offer and Acceptance Program).

The merger should really be an exciting announcement for medical students. They'll have equal access to a vast array of residency programs. MD students are now eligible to apply for many residency positions that once weren't available to them. Transitioning all programs participating in the AOA Match transition to the new system would increase the available first-year residencies by more than 1,200 positions (https://www.hhs.gov).

It's also important to point out that allopathic graduates can complete their residency training at a program that's achieved Osteopathic Recognition (https://www.usmle.org). The ACGME notes that these programs will expect MD graduates to demonstrate knowledge of osteopathic teaching and training, but they can do so in a variety of ways. Graduates may need to have gained experience by completing osteopathic elective rotations, for example. They may even need to complete a structured onboarding program.

While some have expressed concern that DO students will be at a disadvantage without a pool of residencies reserved solely for them, they stand to reap certain benefits. For starters, they no longer must go through two separate application processes to access all the first-year residencies.

Furthermore, students attending osteopathic medical schools don't have to take multiple sets of licensing exams to apply to every program. Previously, DO students needed to complete the United States Medical Licensing Examination (USMLE) series in addition to the Comprehensive Osteopathic Medical Licensing Examination (COMLEX) sequence if they were interested in applying to both DO and MD residency programs. Now, both licensing exams will be equally recognized (https://www.osha.gov).

The advice for all medical students wanting to secure their choice residency program is the same both pre- and post-merger: work hard in school and score as high as possible on licensing exams.

Summary

Residency or postgraduate training is specifically a stage of graduate medical education. It refers to a qualified physician (one who holds the degree of MD, DO, DPM, MBBS, and MBChB) who practices medicine, usually in a hospital or clinic, under the direct or indirect supervision of a senior medical clinician registered in that specialty such as an attending physician or consultant. In many jurisdictions, successful completion of such training is a requirement to obtain an unrestricted license to practice medicine, and in particular, a license to practice a chosen specialty.

An individual engaged in such training may be referred to as a resident, registrar, or trainee, depending on the jurisdiction. Residency training may be followed by fellowship or subspecialty training. While medical school teaches physicians a broad range of medical knowledge, basic clinical skills, and supervised experience practicing medicine in a variety of fields, medical residency gives in-depth training within a specific branch of medicine. This chapter focused on the complexities involved in the postgraduate training of medical graduates and the impact this arduous process can have on the professional life of beginning medical trained physicians.

References

Accreditation Council for Graduate Medical Education. https://www.acgme.org/

American Association Medical Colleges. https://www.aamc.org/

American Medical Association. https://www.ama-assn.org

American Medical Student Association. https://www.amsa.org/

College of Family Physicians of Canada. https://www.cfp.ca/

Colleges of Medicine of South Africa. https://www.cmsa.co.za

Comprehensive Osteopathic Medical Licensing Examination. https://www.nbome.org/assessments/comlex-usa/

Educational Commission for Foreign Medical Graduates. https://www.ecfmg.org

Electronic Residency Application Service. https://students-residents.aamc.org/applying-residencies-eras/applying-residencies-eras

Institute of Medicine. https://nam.edu

Internal Medicine Residency Categorical Program. https://www.massgeneral.org/medicine/internal-medicine/education/residency/categorical

John Hopkins Hospital. https://www.hopkinsmedicine.org/the_johns_hopkins_hospital/

National Resident Matching Program. https://www.nrmp.org

Public Citizen. https://www.citizen.org

Royal College of Physicians and Surgeons. https://www.royalcollege.ca/rcsite/home-e

Supplemental Offer and Acceptance Program

United States Department of Health and Human Services. https://www.hhs.gov

United States Medical Licensing Examination. https://www.usmle.org

United States Occupational Safety and Health Administration. https://www.osha.gov

William Osler. https://en.wikipedia.org/wiki/William_Osler, https://www.nrmp.org/wp-content/uploads/2015/09/SOAP-FAQ-Schools.pdf

William Stewart Halsted. https://en.wikipedia.org/wiki/William_Stewart_Halsted

CHAPTER 4

Health Care in the United States

Status of Health Care in the United States

Overall, in the United States when it comes to how health care is available to its citizens, the mechanisms to deliver it are through a variety of agencies and entities that involve both the private and public sectors including the federal government. Included in the health care system are a variety of health providers consisting of clinics (private, public, and free), hospital-based systems, physician-based practices, and finally insurance companies. Without question, the major impediment regarding the quality of what health care is received in the United States is the cost of that health care. The United States spends more as a percentage of its gross national product than any other major developed country on its health care. Often it is stated that if one focuses on *technology alone*, there is little argument regarding the quality of the health care that can be delivered; however, if one factors the cost of applying that technology, it usually results in access only to those who can afford it through the private sector. If health care coverage is provided through only one provider or in combination with the private and public sectors—such as, insurance companies or government programs, such as, Medicare and Medicaid—health care can be accessible. If the person has served as a member of the country's armed forces, they are afforded the benefit from having served their country of accessing health care through the Veterans Administration (VA). Thus, this government system provides health care for free for those who served in the military; however, the system has been plagued with criticism because of the quality of the health care delivered and the length of time it takes to secure appointments.

The overarching major criticism that has plagued the health care system in the United States when compared to other developed countries is the lack of universal health care coverage for all citizens. There is no universal health care coverage for all the citizens of the United States, although there have been several attempts to enact legislation to create universal coverage. More recently, partial success has been achieved with the approval and implementation of the Affordable Care Act (ACA). Since being enacted, approximately 30 million Americans have now been enrolled for coverage through the ACA, especially those persons who would not have had the opportunity to become covered without the legislation (American Hospital Association, 2016; Rosenthal, 2013). The law creating the ACA has now been upheld by the U.S. Supreme Court no fewer than three times with the most recent ruling taking place on June 17, 2021.

Over the last decade, the percentage of health care spending that has been provided by the United States federal government, that is, through Medicare, Medicaid, the Children's Health Insurance Program, and the VA equaled 64% of the total cost to deliver that care (Department for Professional Employees, 2016; Fisher, 2012). The demographic profile of those insured is usually measured as follows—individuals under the age of 65 most often acquire health insurance usually through two mechanisms: (1) through their own effort or through a family member, both being made available through an employer; or (2) they may need to purchase their health care insurance on their own, perhaps needing assistance to cover the cost of the health care using via a variety of mechanisms; or the worst-case scenario, if they cannot afford the cost, then unfortunately they remain uninsured. This last condition only drives up the cost of health care for all because those unpaid health care expenditures must be covered, and as a result, this generates higher premiums that are paid by those who can afford to pay for their health care. Public sector employees, meaning working for local government agencies, will usually have their health care coverage premiums covered by their employer (Himmelstein & Woolhandler, 2016; Leonard, 2016). Overall, the system of providing health care that is reasonable in its scope, coverage that is universal, and at the same time tries to be affordable created the term "managed care." It is still debatable whether overall managed care can and will be sustainable for the future (*How FEHB Relates to Other Government Health Insurance*, 2017).

Life expectancy in the United States had been 78.6 years calculated from the time of birth back in 1990 (CIA k, 2017; Murray et al., 2013). Unfortunately, since then life expectancy has declined in the country with the reason attributed to the Covid-19 pandemic (Tinker, 2018).

When addressing the quality of the health care delivered in the United States, a study conducted by the U.S. National Institutes of Health (NIH) in 2013 showed that among the 17 high-income countries, the United States had the highest prevalence in the following categories: obesity, motor vehicle accidents, infant mortality, coronary and pulmonary diseases, sexually transmitted diseases, teenage pregnancies, injuries, and homicides (National Research Council and Institute of Medicine, 2013). In comparative terms, evaluating efficiency versus cost, the United States ranked near the bottom because its health care system is most expensive, but at the same time, it has the most undesirable outcomes in terms of access, equity, and importantly efficiency (Fullman et al., 2018; The Commonwealth Fund, 2017).

It has often been suspected that one of the main, if not the primary, reasons explaining why Americans do not access health care on a regular basis is the high cost of health care in the United States (Witters, 2019). However, the impact of the ACA has been demonstrated to have made a difference because the percentage of uninsured Americans has declined since the law was enacted dropping by 5% overall (Witters, 2019). The number of uninsured Americans hovers between 27 and 30 million, a number that compels effort to promoting expansion of the ACA. The number of uninsured has been attributed as one of the leading factors contributing to the country toping the lists of unfavorable categories such as increased in mortality (The Harvard Gazette, 2009). A study conducted at Harvard Medical School reported that the annual deaths saved because of the ACA numbered 65,000 (CNN Politics, 2015). The study also demonstrated a 40% higher mortality rate among those who are uninsured (CNN Politics, 2015).

Importantly for Americans, the ACA that informally came to be known as "Obamacare" after becoming law in 2010 survived multiple court challenges to its legitimacy including a challenge argued in the U.S. Supreme Court in 2015. The law is now affirmed in all 50 states (Thomasson, 2002).

What Should Applicants to Medical School Know About Changes in Health Care?

History

From the historical perspective in the United States, when compared to its European counterparts that have traditionally provided for its citizens a nationalized government supported health care system, health insurance plans were created by and delivered through employers. When it became difficult to attract and/or retain employees, the private sector created a private employment-based system through the Stabilization Act of 1942. The system allowed employers to provide employees with health insurance benefits and health care packages in lieu of higher salaries as a fringe benefit. The market created a private employment-based system. Creation of this system allowed the practice of employer-sponsored health insurance (Thomasson, 2002).

Statistics

Hospitalizations

In the United States in 2022, there were 33.7 million hospital admissions into the nation's medical facilities. From 2019 to 2021 many hospitalizations were attributed to the Covid-pandemic. More than 4,115 people have been hospitalized or died with Covid-19 in the United States, even though they've been fully vaccinated, according to new data from the Centers for Disease Control and Prevention published in 2021 (CNBC, 2021). So far, at least 750 fully vaccinated people have died after contracting Covid, but the CDC noted that 142 of those fatalities were asymptomatic or unrelated to Covid-19, according to data released by the CDC. The CDC received 3,907 reports of people who have been hospitalized with breakthrough Covid infections, despite being fully vaccinated. Of those, more than 1,000 patients were asymptomatic, or their hospitalizations weren't related to Covid-19, according to the CDC (CNBC, 2021).

According to a statistical brief by the Healthcare Cost and Utilization Project, there were 35.7 million hospitalizations in 2016 (https://www.ahrq.gov/data/hcup/index.html), a significant decrease from the 38.6 million in 2011. For every 1,000 in the population, there was an average of 104.2 stays and each stay averaged $11,700, an increase from the $10,400 cost per stay in 2012 (Weiss & Elixhauser, 2012), 7.6% of the population had overnight stays in 2017 (FastStats, 2019), each stay lasting an average of 4.6 days (CNBC, 2021).

A study by the NIH reported that the lifetime per capita expenditure at birth, using year 2000 dollars, showed a large difference between health care costs of females ($361,192) and males ($268,679). A large portion of this cost difference is in the shorter lifespan of men, but even after adjustment for age (assuming men live as long as women), there still is a 20% difference in lifetime health care expenditures (Alemayehu & Warner, 2004).

Health Insurance and Accessibility

As stated previously, the United States, unlike any other developed country in the world, fails to provide basic health care for all its citizens (Institute of Medicine Committee on the Consequences of Uninsurance, 2004). However, most of the population maintains health care coverage through a variety of plans that are basically a combination of state and federal programs working jointly with the private insurance sector (Institute of Medicine Committee on the Consequences of Uninsurance, 2004). According to most recent information (Institute of Medicine, Committee on Monitoring Access to Personal Health Care Services, 1993), health insurance coverage was provided by employers for their employees that covered 56% of Americans, approximately 156 million Americans. Programs provided by the federal government, such as, Medicaid, services 19.3% or 1 out of every 5 or 75 million low-income Americans, followed by Medicare, services 17.2% of the American population or 56 million Americans, along with what has been provided as the result of the ACA, which are referred to health insurance marketplaces, services 22 million Americans, even though there may be issues regarding both access and choosing providers (Institute of Medicine, Committee on Monitoring Access to Personal Health Care Services, 1993). This collective system of various plans still leaves many Americans as uninsured that collectively add to the burden of escalating health care costs, in part, because uninsured individuals, when they are forced to seek medical care, flock to the nation's emergency rooms or urgent treatment centers seeking treatment. The emergency room is the most expensive option, but under the circumstance, it is their only option to seek medical assistance.

Having any number of uninsured citizens is a problem, but it is also significant because it accounts for a significant number of unnecessary deaths in the United States annually (The Commonwealth Fund, 2018). With the implementation of the ACA, it has had an impact on reducing the number of uninsured Americans; therefore, it is reasonable to assume that the numbers of unnecessary deaths will gradually reduce once the ACA becomes more widely available, especially if states agree to expand the number of individuals who would be allowed to enroll in Medicaid.

Another important aspect to the benefits of an increasing population able to secure health care coverage, for example, through the ACA, is the impact it has when factoring together the ability to save lives plus the cost savings incurred as the result of lives saved. Rough estimates have suggested that up to $325,000 in health care costs per patient has been saved because the individual was able to secure health insurance through the ACA (CDC, 2016). Dealing with the overall financial aspect of the benefits of the ACA, it has also helped to prevent personal bankruptcies with almost 25% of seniors reported bankruptcies because of unpaid health care expenses (Docteur & Oxley, 2004).

Global Context of Health Status in the United States

For many categories, such as under-five child mortality, maternal deaths, life expectancy for a child born before 2015, and over-life expectancy, the United States ranks well below the other major developed countries in the word (World Health Statistics, 2016).

Causes of Mortality in the United States

In the United States, the top three causes of death factoring in all ages and both sexes have remained constant over the years. They are cardiovascular diseases, cancer of all types, and neurological disorders including dementia (FastStats, 2017). When examining overall health outcomes and early mortality, the major contributing factors are not related to either communicable or noncommunicable conditions (NPR, 2013).

Facilities

By facilities it means what are the various types of health care available and who operates them. In the United States, many of the facilities are owned and operated by government agencies, whether they be local, city, county, state, and federal governments.

When counting the number of hospital facilities in the United States, there are a total of 6,090 registered facilities with 4,840 listed as community-based facilities. Community-based hospitals comprise nonfederal, short-term, or specialty facilities (Case & Deaton, 2020). Within this list, most of the facilities ~70% are not-for-profit, which includes 20% run by the federal government, with the remaining 30% being privately owned for-profit hospitals. The total admissions in U.S. hospitals for 2021 are 36.2 million and counting. An important piece of federal legislation was enacted in 1946 that called for the federal government to reimburse hospitals for the cost of treating economically disadvantaged patients. Without this support, these hospitals would not be able to sustain themselves financially.

In recent years, there has been an attempt to reduce the overall expense of providing hospital care, especially when it comes to servicing economically disadvantaged patients (Cohen et al., 2017). Differences in available health care facilities have also been predicated based on market size and competition, meaning that local population density often is the determining factor whether local health care facilities can be sustained financially (Glied & Altman, 2017).

Regarding where physicians tend to practice, almost two thirds of physicians are in practice in a group setting consisting of seven or fewer practitioners, with most of these practices owned by physicians; however, there has been a trend over the past several years for physician-based practices to become incorporated into larger based health care systems. Whether this change has improved overall patient care is debatable.

Across the United States, there are no government owned medical facilities available to serve the health care needs of the entire public. On occasion, such as, national disasters, the Defense Department and/or Office of Emergency Management can be called upon to establish field hospitals to help provide emergency care. This condition was a common occurrence during the Covid-19 pandemic of 2020–2021. These facilities are usually staffed with U.S. military personnel such as the National Guard.

The one major hospital system organized and supported financially by the U.S. federal government is the one operated by the Department of Veterans Affairs, known as the VA System. The system was mandated by the U.S. Congress to meet the health care needs of those who served in any branch of the American Armed Forces. Although when originally conceived the focus was to meet the health care needs of those wounded in America's wars; however, over time when the service populations lowered to cause concern whether the VA system could remain sustainable, the qualifying service requirements were expanded to include non-service or war-related injuries. This means health care for these service personnel can be provided through the remaining years of a service person's life regardless of the cause.

Another minor system operated by the federal government, minor in terms of the number of people served, is operated by the Indian Health Service (IHS). The health care system operated by IHS serves only Native Americans with the care provided via contracted services made available to the agency.

At this juncture, a definition of the types of health care facilities that are available for patients is warranted. The function of hospitals is to provide outpatient care through specialty clinics and emergency rooms in addition to their main responsibility, which is to provide in-patient care. An example of a specialty clinic would be a Surgicenter. For patients who are terminally ill (expected to live less than 6 months), there are facilities referred to as Hospice. Facilities that focus on obstetric and gynecologic specialty clinics providing prenatal, family planning, and dysplasia services are usually government-funded. These clinics are usually serviced by nurse practitioners. Clinics that provide emergency care on an outpatient are Urgent Treatment Centers; however, these clinics are not free; nonetheless, patients are treated even if they cannot pay for services rendered.

Although these clinics tend to cover the vast array of patient needs, there is one important patient population that often cannot access any of the clinics listed above. This patient population often consists of individuals who are by description economically disadvantaged, otherwise listed as poor. These special clinics are the "free" clinics. At last count, there are 1,400 free clinics operating in the United States. For those economically disadvantaged, free clinics are the last resort for these individuals to receive basic health care. Those who qualify to receive health care access through free clinics are also individuals who may have become uninsured as the result of becoming unemployed or their income level results in the inability to afford health insurance. Whether it is to receive a flu shot if they are suffering from flu-like symptoms, or the diabetic patient who needs to receive insulin to control their blood sugar levels, or if it is simply vitamins, free clinics fill the void. Free clinics may also provide dental, optical, and pharmacy services. Financial support of not-for-profit free clinics is often a delicate balance of securing funds through donations, fund-raising activities, and grants.

Finally, facilities designed to provide long-term care of patients are referred to as nursing homes or long-term care facilities. These facilities were a cause of concern with respect to the Covid-19 pandemic as these facilities were often the source of pockets of infection that led to many fatalities.

Physicians (MDs and DOs)

The chief practitioner legally responsible for the delivery of health care to patients is the physician. In the United States, the medical education of physicians is a long and arduous process consisting of many years didactic education followed by years of clinical education and training including medical school, residency, and if necessary, fellowships. The training is necessary to eventually acquire a medical license to practice in the state the physician wishes to practice.

Acquiring a medical license requires successful performance of the steps through the United States Medical Licensing Examination (USMLE) system. The first step of the USMLE evaluates whether the medical student can satisfactorily understand and apply the basic science education delivered during the first 2 years of medical school. This material serves as the foundation for the clinical training that will serve as the focus of the remaining 3rd and 4th years of medical school. The subjects that are covered in the Step 1 exam include anatomy, biochemistry, microbiology, pathology, pharmacology, physiology, behavioral sciences, nutrition, genetics, and aging. Step 1 is taken toward the end of the 2nd year of medical school. The Step 2 exam focuses on testing whether medical students can successfully apply their medical knowledge and skills to actual clinical practice as experienced during the medical student's 4th year of study. Next is the Step 3 exam. It is taken after the 1st year of residency has been completed. It is focused on testing whether interns can apply their medical knowledge to the unsupervised practice of medicine.

In the United States, the American College of Physicians defines the term "physician" as anyone who has graduated from an accredited and valid medical school. In the United States, there are two paths to becoming a physician. Individuals can attend either an allopathic medical school graduating with the Doctor of Medicine (MD) degree, or they can attend an "osteopathic" medical school graduating with the Doctor of Osteopathic Medicine (DO) degree. The difference between the two is based upon the following: allopathic medicine focuses on treatment strategies concentrating on the use of pharmaceuticals, that is, drugs to treat diseases, whereas osteopathic trained physicians focus on a holistic, alternative, or complementary medical approach to treat diseases that relies less on the use of drugs as medicines.

Medical Products, Research and Development

The United States is no different than most developed countries of the world when it comes to the production and manufacture of both medical devices and pharmaceuticals. Both commodities require financial support that can be provided by both public and private sources. The total amount of funding amounts to billions of dollars that is divided approximately 60% from the private sector and 40% from public sources. As the result of this public–private partnership, the United States has been the world leader in medical innovation, whether one measures outcomes in terms of new drugs or medical devices approved for human use. Much of the emphasis during the past 5 years is centered in biotechnology. However, one drawback to the growth of this industry in the United States is the high cost of clinical testing in the country, thus driving a greater percentage of clinical trials to be performed outside the United States.

Health Care Provider Employment in the United States

As the cost of health care in the United States continues to increase as a significant percentage of the country's gross domestic product (GDP), the expectation is that this cost will continue to increase at a significant rate greater than inflation (>5%). This is partly due to the retirement of the baby boomers, resulting in an increase in the geriatric population of the country. The cost of providing health care increases 8-fold for individuals who are 45-yr or older compared to individuals below the age of 45. Increases such as these are basically unsustainable for a country, any country, to remain financially solvent.

Alternative Medicine

It was mentioned earlier that the path of becoming a practicing physician can be accomplished by attending either an allopathic or an osteopathic medical school with the difference between the two being for those attending osteopathic medical school learning the practice of medicine through the lens of alternative or complementary medicine (ACM). The list of procedures or techniques acquired by the graduates of osteopathic medical schools include the use of herbal products, massages, energy healing, homeopathy, cryotherapy, transcranial magnetic stimulation, and ultrasound technology. Delivery and implementation of these treatments allow patients to take greater control of their own health allowing patients to treat their chronic symptoms more effectively, in addition, to allowing patients to address their medical conditions through nutritional and social means. One drawback to greater acceptance of these ACM procedures is the fact that many of these procedures are not covered by health insurance, thus decreasing their popularity.

Spending

It has been well-publicized for many years that the United States spends more on health care (several trillion dollars, more than $13K for every man, woman, and child and approaching 20% GDP) than most developed countries, yet for the amount spent the country ranks near the bottom in many key categories used to quantitate efficiency. Factored in this calculation are the costs required to administer, deliver, and utilize the services. In another key barometer used to monitor overall costs, the rate of increase is occurring faster when compared to the rising rate of inflation (Marmor et al., 2009).

Other major factors also affect the affordability of health care in the country. One is the high cost of prescription drugs (Health Costs, 2016). Another is the average cost of certain medical procedures such as the performance of angioplasties, C-sections, and joint replacement surgeries. Certain medical tests such as CT and MRI scans have also contributed to the high cost of care because their use has increased dramatically over the past several years (Pfeffer, 2013). Hospital costs have also increased at rates exceeding inflation often without any clear indication that their efficiency has improved. One indicator that sheds light on this fact has been seen by the length of hospital stays has not appreciably decreased in accordance with the increase in expenditures. Thus, the question is—are we paying more for hospital services for the same quality of care received, yet there has been very little effect on shortening the length of the average hospital stay. On average for every dollar spent in the United States on health care, 31% goes to hospital care, 21% goes to physician/clinical services, 10% to pharmaceuticals, 4% to dental, 6% to assisted living/nursing homes, 3% to home health care, 3% for other retail products, 3% for government public health activities, 7% to administrative costs, 7% to investment, and 6% to other professional services, such as physical therapists, occupational therapists, and optometrists (Health Costs, 2016). With that said, it is also well-documented that in the United States approximately 20% of health care costs are directly linked to the last 3 years of life (Pfeffer, 2013).

Involved Organizations and Institutions

At the federal level in the United States under the Department of Health and Human Services (DHHS), there exists various agencies that have very specific roles and functions with respect to how health care is regulated for its citizens, such as, the Food & Drug Administration (FDA) approves all pharmaceutical produced medications and medical device use including laboratory testing; the Centers for Disease Control (CDC) creates and implements policy designed to protect the health and safety of the country focusing on overall public health; the Agency of Health Care Quality & Research advances excellence in health care by producing evidence safer, higher quality, more accessible, equitable, and affordable health care; the Agency Toxic Substances & Disease Registry, which regulates the waste and disposal of toxic substances; and the NIH performs medical research hopefully to discover cures, if not, then improved ways to effectively treat human diseases.

At the state level, health departments are maintained, while at the local municipality level including counties, one will find branch offices of state health departments. These agencies have the power to execute and regulate state health laws. In several states, health care professionals occupy positions on state boards, while in other states the positions are appointed by the local governor of that state. Federal legislation, such as the McCarran–Ferguson Act, delegates oversight and regulation of health care from the federal government to the states. Per matters related to oversight, health care agency and organizations submit voluntarily to participate in overview conducted by the Joint Commission on Accreditation of

Hospital Organizations. This commission will also conduct oversight on individual physician practices and if sufficient complaints brought against any practicing physician can lead to them losing their license to practice in that state where the alleged violation took place. Finally, the Centers for Medicare and Medicaid Services regulate all assisted living and nursing home facilities in the country.

"Certificates of Need" for Hospitals

Since 1978, the U.S. federal government has required that in the planning to create a new hospital in any given state, the responsible party must first demonstrate to the appropriate state agency, a Certificate of Need. The intent of this policy was to reduce overall health care costs by minimizing the presence of duplication of services in any given local geographical area. It has been argued that the program has led to increased costs as the result of decreasing competition among health facilities (Ho et al., 2009).

Licensing of Providers

One of the most powerful medical associations in existence in the United States that functions to lobby the federal government on all matters related to the delivery of medicine and medical practice, how physicians are educated, trained, and practice in the country is the American Hospital Association (AHA). Since 1910, it has successfully influenced the federal government to limit the number of new physicians to approximately 100,000 per year. This policy has intentionally or unintentionally created a physician shortage in the country (Dalmia, 2009).

However, more impactful has been the success of the AHA to keep physicians as the key component in providing health care services even when there are other qualified health care practitioners available to perform the same procedure without any reduction in the efficiency or quality of the service provided. This has led to the long-standing policy of physicians being paid to perform *procedures* rather than for providing quality *results* (Cauchon, 2005). Another example is the ability to prescribe medications and perform injections, although the recent Covid-19 pandemic created the scenario that allowed other health care professions such as pharmacists, physician assistants, in addition to nurses to administer vaccines.

Quality Assurance

One of the major issues facing health care is determining the quality of the service provided to and for patients. Over time, a plethora of assessment methods have been created to best determine when health care delivered is it the best it can be for the patient. Now with the emphasis on quality of the care delivered by practitioners, an important shift has taken place to address this change, meaning the focus has gradually moved to outcomes assessment with the center of attention now on the practitioner. To ensure participation in this shift of focus to outcomes assessment will mean maintaining quality performance will be directly linked to one's individual personal level of compensation. Another important component of this effort to become more transparent will be the public reporting of performance whether it is hospitals, clinics, or all practitioners regardless of the level of responsibility. It is argued that making such reports public will in the long-term improve the overall quality of health care delivered to and received by patients.

Overall System Effectiveness

How does the United States measure up to the responsibility to deliver quality health care for its citizens?

Measures of Effectiveness

The health care system in the United States unfortunately has had a track record of providing unequal health care services for its citizens. When one considers the country has the scientific expertise and overall resources to create, deliver, develop, invent, and importantly test for efficacy, new medicines, and ways to improve diagnoses, the fact that access to what should be high quality health care available to all, as a right, not as a privilege, regardless of age, gender, ethnicity, and importantly, the capability to pay, is not equal across the socioeconomic spectrum of its citizens.

To provide a level of assessment to determine the quality of care delivered, the U.S. government through the DHHS monitors and evaluates system effectiveness through services provide by researchers and policymakers whose responsibility it is to track deliverables through a system of trends and other measures. DHHS created the Health System Management Project designed to monitor the data collected with respect to the access to, quality of, and the overall cost of the care provided, in concert with monitoring the overall health of the population at large, along with assessing the quality and effectiveness of the entire health care workforce.

Waiting Times

One of the arguments that has been made for years that best defines the effectiveness of the health care system in the United States versus what has been proposed under the heading of "socialized medicine" or "managed care" is the length of time required to obtain appointments. Socialized medicine or managed care has been labeled to be burdened by the length of time required to secure appointments, rightly or wrongly. With that said, it is perceived that certain groups of Americans wait longer for appointments. The percentages listed for wait times for specialist appointments and those for elective surgery are both far less than what times are reported for the same services in other developed countries, such as Canada, France, Germany, the United Kingdom, New Zealand, and Switzerland (Reinhardt, 2008). For citizens of the United States, an appreciable percentage of the wait times incurred can be explained simply by the fact that certain patients may wish to secure appointments with either specific facilities, clinics, and/or practitioners because of choice, not necessarily governed simply by availability regardless of the facility, clinic, and/or practitioner.

Population Health: Quality, Prevention, Vulnerable Populations

Most health policy analysts agree that the effectiveness of any health care system is predicated on the overall health of the citizenry of the country. The healthier a general population is, the longer the lives those individuals will live. There are several measurements that are often used to quantify quality of life issues. They are life expectancy, composite life measurements (time in years when one is expected to be in good to excellent health sometimes referred to as "good or better health, free of activity limitations"). It is generally agreed that the U.S. health care system does not promote a state of "wellness." Teen pregnancy and low birth rates are still an issue in the country. Diseases such as obesity, high-blood pressure, high cholesterol, and type 2 diabetes are practically endemic in the country especially in the Southeast. Although many of these diseases and disease conditions are associated with seniors, what has become alarming to health officials is these health conditions are appearing in younger adults and even more prevalent in youngsters. Health officials are troubled by the fact that the change in health conditions is not associated with an effect across the population but is prevalent in certain ethnic and minority groups versus the general population. Of concern also is the lack of access and availability of health care to those minority populations who often have higher percentages of individuals afflicted with diseases associated with these groups, such as, cardiovascular disease, type 2 diabetes, obesity, high-blood pressure, and colon cancer.

Innovation: Workforce, Healthcare IT, R&D

In the United States, investment in the health care workforce, advances in technology, and research & development new medicines is a key element to maintain the cutting-edge regarding health care. However, significant issues remain with respect to access of these elements to everyone regardless of age, ethnicity, gender, race, or ability to pain.

Compared to Other Countries

As stated previously, the health care system as currently practiced is the most expensive in the world, yet for the cost, the outcomes are still poor in virtually all categories in which assessments are followed especially in terms of access, efficiency, and equity. With respect to life expectancy, as of 2021 the United States ranks 60th in the world, although such rankings now must be modified because of Covid. It ranks 54th in terms of infant mortality. When compared to other countries, Americans undergo cancer screenings, including MRI, and CT scans more than any other developed country. Whether this screening pays dividends in terms of identifying or early detection is a debatable issue. It has also been argued that when comparing similar results from other developed countries, on average upward of 100,000 Americans die; however, if these same people were living in either Australia, France, or Japan, they would not have perished from their illnesses. This attributed to the efficiency of the health care systems, which are so vastly superior to what is found in the United States (Dunham, 2008). Thus, the universal consensus is the United States spends exorbitant amounts of money for its health care, that is, by comparison, one of the worst in the world when factoring outcomes (Case & Deaton, 2020).

Several other factors influence how effective is the American health care system. When analyzed, they clearly show a disproportional effect on patient outcomes when one examines where the health care is delivered, meaning specific geographical areas of the country, in addition to the educational level of patients, and overall general health of the population (Ezzati et al., 2008). Life expectancy is generally lower for women versus men, by as much as 3 years for men and 6 years for women and this trend is especially prevalent in the certain areas of the United States—Appalachia, Deep South, Mississippi Delta, Southern Plains, and Texas (Ezzati et al., 2008). Those whose ages were from 25 to 64 and were by definition "poorly educated" were found to have lower life expectancies compared to educated individuals living in the same area. The difference being attributed to the high propensity to find individuals living with obesity, obsessive smoking, cardiovascular disease, and high blood pressure (Jemal et al., 2008). One cannot discount the overall effect of disparities when factoring in health care outcomes as this population has been historically underserved when it comes to access to quality health care. This factor has been brought to the forefront during the Covid pandemic in so many ways, whether it is access to initially testing for the coronavirus, or contact with health providers when symptomatic, or the availability to receive Covid vaccines or the denial to want to receive vaccination because of a distrust in the health care system in general, all created an environment of a lack of trust in the system.

Health Care Reform and Debate

In America, its citizens have had a divided opinion on evaluating whether the health care system in the country was good versus bad when compared to other countries. Prior to the passing of the ACA, 45% of the population thought that the country's health care was effective versus 39% of the population thought that other countries around the world had better health care system (School of Public Health, 2008).

The focus of the debate that has been the center of the controversy whether universal health care should be a right available for all citizens had at its core whether there should be a single payer providing the care, especially to that population best described as the uninsured (Reynolds, 2002). The debate over whether free-market advocates should have a choice in their purchase of health insurance argue that such control implies government intervention. Since the implication labeled the single payer health care as "socialized medicine," it was not adapted as a key element in the final legislation.

Patient Protection and Affordable Care Act (2010)

The ACT as Public Law 111–148 was signed into law as the major health care legislation by President Barack Obama on March 23, 2010. The major provisions of the law that took effect in 2014 allowed the expansion of Medicaid eligibility for persons with incomes up to 133% of the federal poverty level (Rice, 2010). With the additional provision of subsidizing insurance premiums for individuals and families with incomes up to 400% of the federal poverty limit and capping health expenses up to 9.8% of total costs (The White House, 2017).

One of the major provisions of the legislation called for all health insurance policies sold in the country to have premiums that must be an "out of pocket" expense. Importantly in addition to providing incentives to businesses to start providing health care insurance for its employees, they were required to eliminate denial of health care based on preexisting conditions and to prohibit implementing annual spending caps. In addition, the legislation provides for the basic support of medical research. How the new program was to be paid for called for the implementation of taxes primarily affecting those individuals in the higher tax brackets receiving Medicare; new fees, such as when individuals use tanning bed facilities and on use of medical devices; taxing the pharmaceutical industry; and ways to eliminate waste in the system (Grier, 2010).

Another important component of the ACA legislation was the introduction of a tax penalty on those specific individuals who refuse to obtain health insurance through anyone of the available plans. The only individuals exempt from this tax penalty are those individuals who fall below the federal poverty limit threshold for income (Hadley & Holahan, 2003). The tax penalty was later removed after a challenge in court that was help held by the U.S. Supreme Court. The Congressional Budget Office routinely performs calculations designed to determine how impactful the legislation will be on reducing the federal deficit and in doing so provides important information that allows Congress to tweak the legislation, if necessary, for the program to meet it budgetary obligations (Manchikanti, 2011). One area of the legislation that needs to be addressed is the discrepancy between the cost of health care comparing urban versus rural settings as it is generally acknowledged that health care costs are higher in rural areas than in urban areas (BBC, 2017).

Health Insurance Coverage for Immigrants

A long-standing political debate in the United States is the issue of illegal and/or undocumented immigrants who annually enter the country most often seeking employment and/or escape from oppressive government regimens in their home country, thus they are fearful of their own lives and those of their children (Carrasquillo et al., 2000). Immigrants can receive health benefits under the ACA; however, undocumented immigrants are initially prohibited to do so, it is up to individual states to determine how they will handle this problem of providing access to health care to those undocumented individuals living within their borders (Agrawal & Venkatesh, 2016). It has been the customary practice for undocumented individuals to seek medical attention either from local community health clinics and/or free clinics that operate in those states (coveredca.com).

The "Burn Out" of Physicians—What Is Going On?

The American physician population has been increasingly subjected to changes in the practice of medicine that has contributed to an alarming increase in burnout out amongst this group of practitioners across the country. On a percentage basis the number is twice the percentage based on the total number of practicing physicians compared to the rate experienced in the general population showing job overall dissatisfaction. Based on this information, it has been projected that physician burnout and turnover amounts to $5 billion in value lost and is projected to grow as the result of the Covid pandemic (Berg, 2020).

Physician burnout means an individual who is angry, argumentative, irritable, and impatient, demonstrates increased absenteeism, decreased productivity, and most alarming a decrease in the quality of the medical service they would provide. The rate of burnout has been estimated to account for 44% of 15,000 physicians who completed a series online surveys distributed to 15,000 physicians across the country (Berg, 2020). The survey demonstrated that the group that reported the highest rate of burnout was the 45–54 age group. This was an alarming finding because this age group is best described as the age group that should be the most productive regarding when their clinical productivity should peak, and the group should be economically stable in terms of their financial status. With depression being the main complaint, the major factors contributing to this deteriorating condition were reported to be working conditions such as long hours, less time for personal time such as family, and overall work-life balance issues. Another alarming statistic reported was many as 14% of those surveyed stated they had considered suicide, but only a third of this group sought out treatment for their condition (Berg, 2020).

Based on physician burnout the number of patient safety issues reported has led to poor clinical care and a decrease in patient satisfaction amongst those practitioners, thus they work less hours and are leaving the practice of medicine versus those that do not report such issues. Overall, with the decrease in productivity, in addition, to the increase in turnover has contributed to the expected shortfall in the number of practicing physicians across the country by 2025 by as many as 95,000 (Berg, 2020). No medical specialty or subspeciality is immune to the impact of physician burnout: emergency room physicians, anesthesiologists, radiologists, general internists, family physicians, oncologists, psychiatrists, general surgeons, trauma surgeons, psychiatrists, cardiologists, dermatologists, obstetrician-gynecologists, gastroenterologists, residents, and even medical students (Berg, 2020).

What Is the Projection of Career Options—Will Certain Specialties or Subspecialties Disappear?

It is projected that the United States will experience a shortage of physicians by as many as 122,000 by 2033 as the demand for physicians increases at a faster rate than they can be educated and trained (Commins, 2017). The specific medical fields to experience the greatest need over this time are primary care physicians (55,200) and specialty care physicians (86,700). Specifically, family and internal medicine physicians and psychiatrists are in demand, while it is projected that there will be decreased need for anesthesiologists, cardiologists, dermatologists, and radiologists because of advanced technologies that have allowed less reliance on those specialists.

Because of the Covid pandemic, according to the AHA, American hospitals lost $200 billion dollars from March to June 2020 (Commins, 2017). Driving up hospital costs, a dramatic loss in hospital services produced a significant cancellation of many clinical services and procedures. However, the impact caused by the pandemic is not expected to be sustained, thus allowing hospitals the opportunity to return to providing pre-Covid services.

Summary

There is no doubt one of the major influencing factors that has and will impact the education and training of medical based practitioners, such as, dentists, nurses, nurse practitioners, physicians, physician assistants, etc., across the many disciplines that constitute the medical profession is the status of the health care system in the country. The state of managed care as the prime mechanism of how health care is delivered in the country has evolved with the caveat that a significant portion of the American population remains underserved, with estimates suggesting as many as 40 million uninsured individuals in the country. The impact of this population wanting, needing, and frankly, demanding greater access to affordable health care contributes to the sustained high cost of delivering health care to this population. The establishment of the ACA has helped address this deficiency; however, the system still has issues mainly addressing both affordability and accessibility. It was hoped through expanded health care legislation, specifically through the expansion of Medicare benefits that would allow these conditions to be addressed that would provide dental, optical, and hearing services to those in need; however, gaining the required congressional approval to support the legislation so far has been unsuccessful.

References

Agrawal, P., & Venkatesh, A. K. (2016). Refugee resettlement patterns and state-level health care insurance access in the United States. American Journal of Public Health, 106(4), 662–663. https://doi.org/10.2105/AJPH.2015.303017

Agency for Healthcare Research and Quality. Healthcare Costs & Utilization Project. https://www.ahrq.gov/data/hcup/index.html

Alemayehu, B., & Warner, K. E. (2004). The lifetime distribution of health care costs. Health Services Research, 39(3), 627–642. https://doi.org/10.1111/j.1475-6773.2004.00248.x

American Hospital Association. (2016, December 1). Fast facts on US hospitals. AHA.org.

BBC. (2017, May 4). Trump health bill: Winners and losers. BBC News.

Berg, S. (2020, January 21). Physician burnout: Which medical specialties feel the most stress. American Medical Association, *Physician Health*.

Carrasquillo, O., Carrasquillo, A. I., & Shea, S. (2000). Health insurance coverage of immigrants living in the United States: Differences by citizenship status and country of origin. American Journal of Public Health, 90(6), 917–923. https://doi.org/10.2105/AJPH.90.6.917

Case, A., & Deaton, A. (2020). Deaths of despair and the future of capitalism. Princeton University Press. p. ix. ISBN 978-0691217079.

Cauchon, D. (2005, March 2) Medical miscalculation creates doctor shortage, USA Today.

CDC. (2016). *National Center for Health Statistics*. Cdc.gov.

CIA k. (2017). County comparison: Life expectancy at birth. CIA.gov. The World Factbook.

CNN Politics. (2015, June 25). *Obamacare lives on after Supreme Court ruling*. CNNPolitics.com.

Cohen, G. R., Jones, D. J., Heeringa, J., Barrett, K., Furukawa, M. F., Miller, D., Mutti, A., James, D. R., Machta, R., Shortell, S. M., Fraze, T., & Rich, E. (2017, December). Leveraging diverse data sources to identify and describe U.S. health care delivery systems, eGEMs, 5(3), 9. https://doi.org/10.5334/egems.200

Commins, J. (2017, June 7). Why compensation for some medical specialties is on the decline. *Healthleaders*.

Dalmia, S. (2009, August 26). The evil-mongering of the American Medical Association. *Forbes*.

Department for Professional Employees. The U.S. health care system: An international perspective—DPEAFLCIO. 2016 Fact Sheet. Dpeaflicio.org

Docteur, E., & Oxley, H. (2004). Health-care systems reform: Lessons from experience. Towards high-performing health systems: Policy studies. The OECD Health Project. OECD. pp. 25, 74. ISBN 978-92-64-01559-3.

Dunham, W. (2008, January 8). France best, U.S. worst in preventable death ranking. Reuters.

Ezzati, M., Friedman, A. B., Kulkarni, S. C., & Murray, C. J. (2008). The reversal of fortunes: Trends in county mortality and cross-county mortality disparities in the United States. The reversal of fortunes: Trends in county mortality and cross-county mortality disparities in the United States. PLOS Medicine, 5(4), e66. https://doi.org/10.1371/journal.pmed.0050066

"FastStats," www.cdc.gov. August 3, 2017.

"FastStats," www.cdc.gov. September 4, 2019.

Fisher, M. (2012). Here's a map of the countries that provide universal health care (America's still not on it). The Atlantic.

Fullman, N., Yearwood, J., Abay, S. M., Abbafati, C., Abd-Allah, F., Abdela, J., et al. (GBD 2016 Healthcare Access and Quality Collaborators). (2018). Measuring performance on the Healthcare Access and Quality Index for 195 countries and territories and selected subnational locations: A systematic analysis from the Global Burden of Disease Study 2016. *Lancet*, 391(10136), 2236–2271. https://doi.org/10.1016/S0140-6736(18)30994-2

Glied, S. A., & Altman, S. H. (2017, September 20). Boosting competition among hospitals, health systems will improve health care. STAT.

Grier, P. (2010, March 21). Health care reform bill 101: Who will pay for reform? Christian Science Monitor.

Hadley, J., & Holahan, J. (2003). Is health care spending higher under Medicaid or private insurance? Inquiry, 40(4), 323–342. https://doi.org/10.5034/inquiryjrnl_40.4.323

"Health Costs." Kaiseredu.org. The Henry J. Kaiser Family Foundation. October 3, 2016. https://www.kff.org

"Health Insurance for Immigrants." Covered California. coveredca.com. November 17, 2016.

Health & Science. CNBC, June 25, 2021.

Himmelstein, D. U., & Woolhandler, S. (2016). The current and projected taxpayer shares of US health costs. *American Journal of Public Health*, 106(3), 449–452. https://doi.org/10.2105/AJPH.2015.302997.

Ho, V., Ku-Goto, M. H., & Jollis, J. G. (2009). Certificate of Need (CON) for cardiac care: Controversy over the contributions of CON. Health Services Research, 44(2 Pt 1), 483–500. https://doi.org/10.1111/j.1475-6773.2008.00933.x

How FEHB Relates to Other Government Health Insurance. FED week. May 25, 2017. https://www.fedweek.com/retirement-financial-planning/fehb-relates-government-health-insurance/

Institute of Medicine, Committee on Monitoring Access to Personal Health Care Services. (1993). Access to health care in America. In M. Millman (Ed.). National Academies Press.

Institute of Medicine Committee on the Consequences of Uninsurance. (2004). Insuring America's health: Principles and recommendations. National Academies Press. p. 25, ISBN 978-0-309-52826-9.

Jemal, A., Ward, E., Anderson, R. N., Murray, T., & Thun, M. J. (2008). Widening of socioeconomic inequalities in the U.S. death rates, 1993–2001. PLoS ONE, 3(5), e2181.

Leonard, K. (2016, January 22). *Could universal health care save U.S. taxpayers money?* U.S. News & World Report.

Manchikanti, L. (2011). Patient Protection and Affordable Care Act of 2010: Reforming the health care reform for the new decade. Pain Physician, 14(1), E35–E67. https://doi.org/10.36076/ppj.2011/14/E35

Marmor, T., Oberlander, J., & White, J. (2009). The Obama administration's options for health care cost control: Hope versus realty. Annals of Internal Medicine, 150(7), 485–489. https://doi.org/10.7326/0003-4819-150-7-200904070-00114

Murray, C. J., Atkinson, C., Bhalla, K., Birbeck, G., Burstein, R., Chou, D., et al. (2013). The state of US health, 1990–2010: Burden of diseases, injuries, and risk factors. JAMA, 310(6), 591–608. https://doi.org/10.1001/jama.2013.13805

National Research Council and Institute of Medicine. (2013). U.S. health in international perspective: Shorter lives, poorer health. Panel on understanding cross-national health differences among high-income countries, In S. H. Woolf & L. Aron (Eds.), Committee on Population, Division of Behavioral and Social Sciences and Education, and Board on Population Health and Public Health Practice, Institute of Medicine. The National Academies Press.

NPR. (2013, January 9). *U.S. Ranks Below 16 Other Rich Countries in Health Report.* Npr.org.

Pfeffer, J. (2013, April 10). The Reason health care is so expensive: Insurance companies. Bloomberg News.

Reinhardt, U. E. (2008, November 21). Why does U.S. health care cost so much? (Part II: Indefensible administrative costs). The New York Times.

Reynolds, A. (2002, October 3). No human insurance? So what? The Cato Institute. Archived from on October 3, 2002.

Rice, S. (2010, March 25). 5 Key things to remember about health care reform. CNN.

Rosenthal, E. (2013, December 21) News analysis-health care's road to ruin. The New York Times

School of Public Health. (2008, March 20). Most republicans think the U.S. Health Care System is the best in the world. Democrats disagree, Press Disagree. Harvard School of Public Health and Harris Interactive.

The Commonwealth Fund. (2017, June 14). Mirror, Mirror 2017: *International Comparison Reflects Flaws and Opportunities for Better U.S. Health Care.*

The Commonwealth Fund. (2018, November 25). *The decline of employer-sponsored health insurance.* Commonwealthfund.org.

The Harvard Gazette. (2009, September 17). *New study finds 45,000 deaths annually linked to lack of health coverage.* Harvard University.

The White House. (2017, February 8). Policies to improve affordability and accountability. whitehouse.gov.

Thomasson, M. A. (2002). From sickness to health: The twentieth-century development of U.S. health insurance. *Explorations in Economic History*, 39(3), 233–253. https://doi.org/10.1006/exeh.2002.0788

Tinker, B. (2018, February 28). *U.S. life expectancy drops for second year in a row.* CNN.

Weiss, A. J., & Elixhauser, A. (2012). Overview of hospital stays in the United States, 2012: Statistical Brief #180. Healthcare Cost and Utilization Project (HCUP) Statistical Briefs. Agency for Healthcare Research and Quality (US).

Witters, D. (2019). U.S. uninsured rate rises to four-year high. Gallup News: Well-being. https://news.gallup.com/poll/246134/uninsured-rate-rises-four-year-high.aspx

World Health Statistics 2016: Monitoring health for the SDGs, sustainable development goals. Annex B, Tables of health statistics by country, WHO region, and globally. World Health Organization. https://www.who.int/docs/default-source/gho-documents/world-health-statistic-reports/world-heatlth-statistics-2016.pdf

PART II

THE DENTAL SCHOOL APPLICANT

CHAPTER 5

The Road to Dental School

Anna Foster Crowe

What Is Dentistry and What Is the American Dental Association?

The American Dental Association, commonly known as the ADA, is a professional organization for future and present members of the dental profession in the United States. Their mission is to "[foster] the success of a diverse membership and [advance] the oral health of the public" (American Dental Association, 2021a). The ADA provides a comprehensive definition of the concept of dentistry. In 1997, the ADA House of Delegates adopted the following definition of dentistry:

> Dentistry is defined as the evaluation, diagnosis, prevention and/or treatment (nonsurgical, surgical or related procedures) of diseases, disorders and/or conditions of the oral cavity, maxillofacial area and/or the adjacent and associated structures and their impact on the human body; provided by a dentist, within the scope of his/her education, training, and experience, in accordance with the ethics of the profession and applicable law (American Dental Association, 2013).

Most people outside of the field would say dentists just treat teeth. While that might be true, there's so much more to dentistry than just the mouth! Dentists are detectives, diagnosticians, surgeons, anatomists, and more, all within one profession.

In the field of health care, dentists are often referred to as doctors of the head and neck. This statement isn't an attempt to encroach on the territory of otolaryngologists, but rather to acknowledge the extensive knowledge and comprehensive training dentists have, not only regarding the teeth but also concerning the entire oral cavity, as well as every organ, muscle, nerve, and blood vessel found above the shoulders. Although most dental schools have moved toward more field-focused curricula overall, many dentists completed their 1st- and 2nd-year didactic courses alongside medical students.

Dentistry and medicine have many similarities, but their differences must not go unnoticed. We'll learn more about the process of being admitted to dental school in Chapter 6, but it's necessary to state that the process is separate from that of medical school. Like many of the other professional health care disciplines, dental schools in America have their own distinctive degree programs. There are two-degree programs offered by accredited dental schools in the United States. Both degrees are achieved through identical curricula and academic requirements. Many dental schools in the country offer a Doctor of Dental Surgery (DDS) degree, while some award a Doctor of Dental Medicine (DMD) degree to their graduates. There are currently 67 dental schools that have been granted accreditation by the Commission on Dental

Accreditation (CODA; National Commission on Recognition of Dental Specialties and Certifying Boards, 2021).

The dental profession has its own unique schooling course, but it also is unique in the sense that not all graduates must complete a residency or internship after graduating. Most general dentists can start practicing once they've passed their licensure examinations. Dental students are expected to pass all educational, written, and clinical examinations to receive their degree and begin practicing as a general dentist, along with possible additional requirements that can vary from state to state (American Dental Association, 2021b). However, many students find themselves drawn to certain specialties in dentistry. Although choosing a specialty is not a necessity in the dental profession like it might be considered in medicine, it is extremely common and there are several specialties within the dental profession. A list of the dental specialties recognized by the American Dental Association's National Commission on Recognition of Dental Specialties and Certifying Boards can be seen below (American Dental Education Association: The Voice of Dental Education, 2021a):

Dental Anesthesiology

Dental Public Health

Endodontics

Oral and Maxillofacial Pathology

Oral and Maxillofacial Radiology

Oral and Maxillofacial Surgery

Oral Medicine

Orofacial Pain

Orthodontics and Dentofacial Orthopedics

Pediatric Dentistry

Periodontics

Prosthodontics

Every general dentist will usually do a little bit of each of these things in practice; however, by the end of their final year, some students feel as though their talents could be best used in a more specialized field. Although many dental students will go on to specialize after dental school, it is always stressed to prospective dental students not to enter school with a laser focus on one single specific area. Many students credit their orthodontists for sparking their love of dentistry in the first place or feeling incredibly drawn to the idea of working with children. Neither of those things is inherently bad, but every person starting dental school needs to understand that the curriculum is going to lay a strong foundation in every area of dentistry. Abscessed teeth and cadaver lab don't make it on many people's list of Top 10 Favorite Things, but even an orthodontist must learn how to prep a tooth in the beginning, even if they won't ever place a single restoration in practice. Being a doctor means mastering all of it, regardless of what you won't use if you end up specializing.

While it's important for dental students to learn the basics of every specialty, it is also important for prospective students to have general knowledge about what each specialist does daily! Dental schools put a lot of emphasis on shadowing for this reason. Admission offices want to see a commitment to the profession, which can be exhibited by spending time in dental offices and observing as many of the specialties as possible. A working knowledge of the basics of each specialized field when applying to dental school is imperative, not only to appreciate the full scope of the field but also to understand all the destinations to which dentistry as a path can lead.

Dental Anesthesiology

Dental anesthesiology is a newer specialty focusing on reducing pain and anxiety in dental patients. It's no secret that some people fear going to the dentist. However, some patients feel a very intense fear that manifests as something often referred to as "dental anxiety." Performing any procedure on a nervous or fearful patient can be extremely difficult for the operator and very traumatic for the patient. This is where dental anesthesiologists come in. Whether they're operating out of a private practice, traveling to multiple offices, or working in a hospital, dental anesthesiologists can provide relief to their patients through sedation and anesthesia, as well as other methods of anxiety and pain management. Many clinicians, such as oral surgeons, feel comfortable administering sedatives and systemic anesthetics for their own procedures. However, dental anesthesiologists are often hired by health care providers without proper experience or certification or when the case is more complex. Ultimately, a dental anesthesiologist's main purpose is to keep patients safe during dental procedures. The programs available in the United States require a DDS or DMD degree, or an equivalent degree from another country, and take 36 months to complete (American Dental Education Association: The Voice of Dental Education, 2021a).

Dental Public Health

Dental public health is one of the less clinical postgraduate paths. Public health focuses on prevention and community outreach efforts to benefit the overall health of the public (which could be assumed from the name). A position in public health is more focused on education, implementing plans and policies, and researching new ways to fight dental diseases in the community (American Dental Education Association: The Voice of Dental Education, 2021a). Generally being outside of the typical dental office environment, this field looks more unique than a typical residency. The programs look different too and vary in many ways. Although different programs have different requirements and lengths, on average a newly graduated dentist is looking at about 14 more months of continuing education courses, which can lead to a certificate, a master's degree, or even an additional Doctorate. There are currently 15 programs in the United States (American Dental Education Association: The Voice of Dental Education, 2021a).

Endodontics

Endodontists are concerned with the internal structures of the tooth, as well as the apices of the roots and the surrounding areas. For this reason, root canal therapy (also known as endodontic treatment) is an endodontist's bread and butter. During this procedure, endodontists remove infected pulp tissue from inside a dead or dying tooth, clean and shape the root canal(s), fill them with a rubbery material, and cap it off with a restoration! This type of therapy relieves the patient's pain and gives the tooth a second chance. Endodontists are in the business of rehabilitating teeth that other clinicians may say are too far gone to save. An endodontic residency program will last an average of 26 months and there are 55 programs in the United States (American Dental Education Association: The Voice of Dental Education, 2021a).

Oral and Maxillofacial Pathology

When asked to quickly name a disease affecting the head and neck, caries would more than likely be the first answer to come to mind for many dental clinicians. However, oral pathologists might have other ideas! Oral and maxillofacial pathology is generally concerned with the diagnosis and treatment of ailments of the oral and maxillofacial areas of the human body. Clinicians in this field might use several different methods of identification, such as observing histological samples acquired through biopsies and examining radiographs. A well-trained pathologist can make a significant difference in patients facing serious maladies. It takes 37 months to become a certified oral and maxillofacial pathologist. There are currently 14 programs in the United States (American Dental Education Association: The Voice of Dental Education, 2021a).

Oral and Maxillofacial Radiology

Oral and maxillofacial radiology is a specialty focused on the constantly evolving technologies and methods used in radiographic imaging of the oral and maxillofacial regions. Not only are they well-versed in the mechanisms of radiographic imaging, but they also stay up to date on important safety guidelines and infection control recommendations to keep patients and clinicians safe. Oral and maxillofacial radiologists are an invaluable resource in dental education and practice. From periapical radiographs captured on intraoral phosphor plates to cone beam computed tomography scans, these dental professionals are trained and expected to be the experts in all things concerning radiographic imaging, be it technique or interpretation. Oral and maxillofacial radiologists will train anywhere from 2 to 3 years at one of the nine programs offered in the United States today (American Dental Education Association: The Voice of Dental Education, 2021a).

Oral and Maxillofacial Surgery

Oral and maxillofacial surgeons must endure a long and challenging program to earn their prestigious titles. The programs in the United States last anywhere from 4 to 6 years and provide training in several different areas to prepare these clinicians for the many scenarios they will face in practice. Although many oral and maxillofacial surgeons stick mostly to third molar extractions once they complete their program, they are capable of handling developmental deformities, traumatic injuries, cancerous lesions, dental implant cases, cosmetic surgeries, and several other conditions. Therefore, many of the 101 programs here in the United States have started offering Doctor of Medicine (MD) degrees to those completing this incredibly rigorous journey (American Dental Education Association: The Voice of Dental Education, 2021a).

Oral Medicine

Oral medicine is one of the newer dental specialties, only becoming recognized by the National Commission on Recognition of Dental Specialties and Certifying Boards on March 2, 2020 (American Dental Association, 2020). Specialists in this field can expect to treat patients that are more medically complex and help manage medically related oral and maxillofacial ailments. Although the field is clinically based, they rarely perform complex surgery and spend a lot of time performing diagnostic procedures. Some programs may require the completion of an advanced education in dentistry or a general practice residency (GPR) program prior to enrollment. There are six currently recognized programs that vary from 2 to 3 years in length. There are also some longer programs that grant master's and PhD degrees upon completion (American Dental Education Association: The Voice of Dental Education, 2021a).

Orofacial Pain

The newest specialty, with its official recognition following oral medicine's recognition by a mere 29 days, is orofacial pain. Orofacial pain largely encompasses the diagnosis and treatment of painful disorders of the head and neck. The disorders include, but are not limited to, disorders of the temporomandibular joint and jaw, different neuropathies, neurovascular pain, headaches, and migraines, as well as sleep disorders (The American College of Prosthodontics, 2017). Although dental schools give their students limited training in the management of all these ailments, these one- to three-year programs will provide a dentist mastery in the specific area of pain in the oral and maxillofacial regions. Twelve programs are currently recognized; however, like oral medicine, they may not all be currently accepting new applicants (American Dental Education Association: The Voice of Dental Education, 2021b).

Orthodontics and Dentofacial Orthopedics

Orthodontics and dentofacial orthopedics, more commonly referred to as simply "orthodontics," is one of the more familiar specialties to the common layperson. If one was privileged enough to have braces as an adolescent, they probably think of their orthodontist as a miracle worker (even if they weren't too happy about it at the time). Orthodontists are known for straightening pearly whites, but they also help patients gain normal oral function and class I, or normal, occlusion! Orthodontics is a highly sought-after specialty due to its ability to be both incredibly lucrative and rewarding. Admission to an orthodontics program requires top grades, as do many other specialties, due to its competitiveness and the fact that there are currently only 67 programs in the United States. The programs can take anywhere from 24 to 36 months to complete (American Dental Education Association: The Voice of Dental Education, 2021a).

Pediatric Dentistry

Most people have seen a pediatric dentist at one point or another since children's teeth are different from adults' teeth. Although students are trained to work with pediatric patients and many general dentists feel comfortable treating children, pediatric dentists are specially trained to deal with young patients, as well as patients who may not be developmentally matched to their age. Young children and patients with special needs are more likely to struggle behaviorally at the dentist due to fear or lack of understanding. Many advanced education programs are emerging to give dentists exposure to special needs programs, but many pediatric programs have this training built into their curricula already. There are 82 programs in the United States currently offering special training to provide dental care to these specific populations. These programs generally last anywhere from 2 to 3 years (American Dental Education Association: The Voice of Dental Education, 2021a).

Periodontics

Periodontics comes from the Greek words meaning "around tooth." The surrounding tooth structures include the gingiva, oral mucosa, bone, periodontal ligaments, and vasculature. Periodontists are ultimately concerned with the health of these structures, or periodontal health, but also place and repair dental implants. Periodontics is an important discipline because about 50% of American adults have periodontal disease and the risk only increases with age. Periodontal disease also disproportionately affects those living in poverty and smokers (Centers for Disease Control and Prevention, 2013). To become a periodontist, one must complete a program lasting around 3 years. There are currently 57 of these programs in the United States (American Dental Education Association: The Voice of Dental Education, 2021a).

Prosthodontics

Prosthodontists are a lot like orthodontists in the sense that their ultimate purpose is to help patients regain oral function. However, in most cases, their patients are missing quite a lot of teeth! Prosthodontists create custom restorations and appliances that can either stay put or be removed. Whether a patient is missing one tooth or all 32, a prosthodontist can help restore function to the mouth using crowns, bridges, and dentures. General dentists often refer their more complex cases to prosthodontists. Prosthodontic training may take up to 3 years. There are 47 prosthodontic programs currently in the United States (American Dental Education Association: The Voice of Dental Education, 2021a).

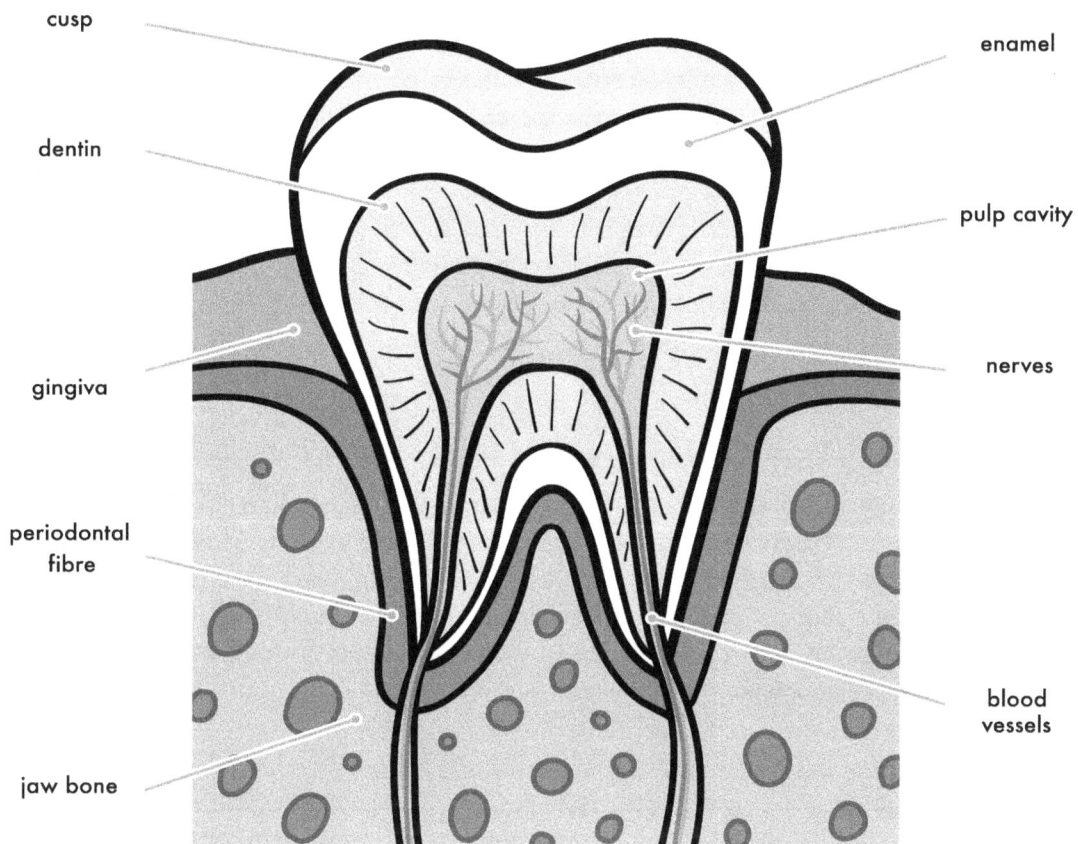

Figure 5.1   Basic components of a tooth and surrounding tissue.

Another common route taken by dentists after graduating from dental school is an Advanced Education in General Dentistry or a GPR program. There are hundreds of programs like these across the United States and they usually take only about a year to complete. These programs can be a great way to sharpen your skills before practicing on your own or an invaluable opportunity to learn more challenging or advanced procedures under the watchful eye of more experienced attendings (Commission on Dental Accreditation, 2021). There is also a plethora of opportunities for dental professionals to participate in less involved continuing education courses in several different, exciting areas, ranging from administering Botox to placing implants to treating sleep apnea.

Aside from the specialty programs and continuing education courses, there are also newer residencies that have yet to be officially recognized by the National Commission on Recognition of Dental

Specialties and Certifying Boards, like residency programs in digital dentistry! The American College of Prosthodontics recently launched a pilot curriculum in digital dentistry at five dental institutions in 2017 (Dentistry Today, 2020). Several additional programs have been launched at other institutions since. The newly recognized specialties by the National Commission on Recognition of Dental Specialties and Certifying Boards, along with the up-and-coming programs in digital dentistry and other exciting fields, prove that dentistry is constantly evolving and exceedingly previously set standards every day.

As you can see, trying to define dentistry in simple terms is impossible! There are so many facets and branches within this complex and exciting field. Let's continue exploring the endless possibilities of a career in dentistry as we head into our next chapter, *Review of the Dental School Application Process*, and begin to understand what all goes into that first step in the wide world of dentistry—the dental school application process.

Summary

The practice of dentistry has long been recognized as an important component of the overall concept of providing health care with attention focused on oral health. The oral cavity has long been recognized as the "portal" through which pathogens can enter the body to induce disease processes that can harm the body's physiological systems. Consequently, having a full complement of teeth, gums, and associated structures is necessary to maintain optimal function of dental systems. This chapter addresses what is involved in dentistry, its components, and sub-disciplines.

References

American Dental Association. (2013). Understanding organized dentistry: A guide for dental schools and dental students. Retrieved from https://www.ada.org/~/media/ADA/Education%20and%20Careers/Files/resources_organized.pdf?la=en

American Dental Association. (2020). Oral medicine recognized as a dental specialty. Retrieved from https://www.ada.org/en/publications/ada-news/2020-archive/march/oral-medicine-recognized-as-a-dental-specialty

American Dental Association. (2021a). General dentistry and interest areas. Retrieved from https://www.ada.org/~/media/ADA/Education%20and%20Careers/Files/resources_organized.pdf?la=en

American Dental Association. (2021b). State licensure for US dentists. Retrieved from https://www.ada.org/en/education-careers/licensure/state-dental-licensure-for-us-dentists#:~:text=The%20educational%20

American Dental Education Association: The Voice of Dental Education (2021a). Advanced education in general dentistry. Retrieved from https://www.adea.org/GoDental/Career_Options/Advanced_Education_in_General_Dentistry.aspx

American Dental Education Association: The Voice of Dental Education (2021b). Advanced dental education programs. Retrieved from https://www.adea.org/GoDental/Career_Options/Advanced_Dental_Education_Programs.aspx

National Commission on Recognition of Dental Specialties and Certifying Boards (2021). Recognized dental specialties: Specialty definitions. Retrieved from https://www.ada.org/en/ncrdscb/dental-specialties/specialty-definitions

Centers of Disease Control and Prevention (2013). Oral health: Periodontal disease. Retrieved from https://www.cdc.gov/oralhealth/conditions/periodontal-disease.html

Commission on Dental Accreditation (2021). Dental programs. Retrieved from https://www.ada.org/en/coda/find-a-program/search-dental-programs#t=us&sort=%40codastatecitysort%20ascending&f:@codatypesubl_coveofacets_0=[Predoctoral%20(DDS%2FDMD)%20Dental%20Education%20Programs]&f:coveo3098a565=[United%20States]

Dentistry Today (2020). ADA recognizes orofacial pain as dentistry's twelfth specialty. Retrieved from dentistrytoday.com/news/todays-dental-news/item/6518-ada-recognizes-orofacial-pain-as-dentistry-s-twelfth-specialty

The American College of Prosthodontics (2017). ACP launches digital dentistry curriculum with partner schools. Retrieved from https://www.dentistrytoday.com/news/todays-dental-news/item/2242-acp-launches-digital-dentistry-curriculum-with-partner-schools

CHAPTER 6

Review of the Dental School Application Process

Anna Foster Crowe

If you've gotten this far, your interest has probably been piqued, and now that you know all the place's dentistry can take you, you're probably asking yourself: *So, how do I take that first step?*

In the United States, the path to dental school is mostly straightforward. Below is a checklist of things you must consider as you begin the application process:

Pick an undergraduate major.

Complete all required academic prerequisite courses.

Take the Dental Admission Test

Complete your application through the Associated American Dental Schools Application Service (AADSAS)

Take advantage of shadowing opportunities with local dental healthcare providers

Serve your community.

Participate in academic research.

Develop your manual dexterity.

Increase your knowledge about professional dental programs through educational opportunities and personal research.

Apply when you feel you are a prepared and complete candidate.

Secure interview invitations and prepare.

Wait patiently for decision day (American Dental Education Association: The Voice of Dental Education, 2021c)

This list may seem daunting, but with proper time management, planning, and dedication, these steps can help lead you where you want to go. Let's talk about each step-in detail.

Undergraduate Education and Major

To be eligible to attend dental school in the United States, one must complete some form of undergraduate program at an accredited university or college. Most dental students possess a 4-year degree or more when matriculating; however, some schools offer hybrid programs that only require the completion of 2–3 years of undergraduate coursework before granting early admission to students that meet the program's expectations (American Dental Education Association: The Voice of Dental Education, 2021g). Whatever your path, you will have to participate in several years of postsecondary education before officially embarking on your dental education.

During your undergraduate program, you'll need to pick a field of study. Many applicants believe they must major in some form of science, but this is not the case. Students pursue plenty of other degrees and most dental schools make it abundantly clear that major choice does not have any effect on their admission decisions. When picking your major, it is important to choose something you enjoy that you know you can excel in. While science majors may have an easier time fitting the required prerequisite courses into their schedule due to overlap in their curricula, musical theatre majors can spare themselves a semester of plant biology and spend their college days singing Sondheim. If they can rattle off molecular weights as fast as they can every color in Joseph's amazing technicolor dream coat, they'll be every bit as successful as any chemistry major!

More and more schools are searching for applicants with well-rounded experiences. Grades and test scores are still important; however, dental schools want to know their students shine in every realm, not just the classroom! Therefore, picking a field of study that truly appeals to you cannot only show admissions offices that you have varied interests but also make the road to dental school a little more enjoyable (American Dental Education Association: The Voice of Dental Education, 2021d).

Prerequisite Courses

As far as prerequisite courses go, it can be difficult to give prospective students a clear-cut checklist of every course that needs to be completed. Each institution has different expectations for its applicants and has different courses that need to be completed prior to admission.

Generally, a student hoping to apply to dental school can expect to take courses in the basic laboratory sciences, such as Biology, Chemistry, and Organic Chemistry, as well as courses in English and Mathematics. All these courses are also extensively tested in their own respective sections on the Dental Admission Test. Many schools also require or recommend that prospective students complete additional courses in Physics, Biochemistry, Microbiology, Anatomy, Physiology, and Cellular Biology. Some examples of other recommended upper-level science course subjects include (but are not limited to) Histology, Immunology, Genetics, Molecular Biology, and Zoology.

Because dental schools are looking for well-rounded applicants, they often appreciate when applicants branch out and take courses that fall within other disciplines, like the arts and humanities. Many social sciences, like Psychology and Sociology, are highly recommended and even required by some schools (American Dental Education Association: The Voice of Dental Education, 2021b)! It makes sense that dental schools want to make sure that the future student doctors they are accepting know how to work well with people since they will be serving the school's patient population and the local community when they matriculate.

Prerequisite requirements vary from institution to institution and can change from time to time, so the best way to stay up to date on different dental schools' requirements is by consulting the AADSAS application or resources provided by the particular school. Students need to plan not only on completing these courses but also on doing well in them! Overall grade point average, as well as science grade point average, will be considered. In fact, your grade point average will be broken down in a myriad of ways for the admissions offices by the AADSAS application, so every class counts. Make every effort to excel in all your academic endeavors, not just the prerequisites.

The Dental Admission Test

One of the most important academic endeavors to consider in applying, besides undergraduate coursework, is the Dental Admission Test, often referred to as the DAT. The DAT is a computer-based multiple-choice exam administered daily at thousands of different prometric exam centers across the country (American Dental Association, 2021c). It is generally recommended that students take the DAT when they have finished all prerequisite coursework since much of the material presented in those classes will be tested on the examination. The test is associated with a fee close to $500, can take up to 5 hours to complete, and is required for admission by every single dental school in the United States; so, anyone considering applying to take the DAT should first read the most up-to-date DAT Guide (American Dental Association, 2021a). This guide is always available on the American Dental Association's website.

A prospective student must register for a DENTPIN, or a Dental Personal Identifier Number, before submitting their testing application. The information connected to the test-takers DENTPIN must match the information on the identification they provide on test day, or else they will not be permitted to participate in the exam and will not be refunded their testing fee. This means they will have to submit a new application, set up a new appointment, and repay the fee. The DENTPIN is connected to the test-taker's dental school application and is used to verify and connect their DAT results to their application. This DENTPIN will also be used for licensure exams once in school and will help identify you to several national dental associations, so keep it handy.

Once you have registered for your DENTPIN, you are ready to apply to take the DAT. Each application expires after 6 months, so be aware of the delicate timeline. You, of course, do not want to apply too late since your application needs to be approved and testing appointments tend to fill up quickly. However, applying too early might give you a false sense of security and leave you with a fast-approaching deadline to complete your exam before you are adequately prepared. Either way, you can end up in a sticky situation and spend way more money than you planned, whether you must purchase a plane ticket to fly to an available appointment slot or reapply because you overestimated your ability to quickly learn the vast amount of material you will be tested on. Due to the demand for appointments and strict time constraints, you need to practice proper time management and planning to ensure you find a suitable date at a nearby location while still providing yourself with adequate study time. The application period can be extended a mere 45 days for a fee and there is always the option to pay to reschedule or even cancel the exam appointment if needed, but it is ultimately easier on you (and your wallet) to just pay the application fee once and book an examination period for which you are most prepared.

Although a prospective student can submit as many applications as they can afford, unfortunately, a test-taker can only actually take the exam itself once every 90 days. After three attempts, the 90-day period is extended to 12 months and the prospective student must request special permission in writing to the American Dental Association to schedule an additional exam date. All these little rules and regulations can seem daunting, but many people who have found themselves in situations like these have also found themselves matriculating into dental school, so do not be discouraged! Just make sure to put forth your best effort and always read the fine print.

The test itself can be broken down into four major sections: Survey of Natural Sciences (which contains all questions concerning the subjects of Biology, General Chemistry, and Organic Chemistry), Perceptual Ability Test (also known as PAT), Reading Comprehension Test, and Quantitative Reasoning Test. There are three optional sections: an optional 15-min tutorial of the testing software at the beginning, an optional 15-min posttest survey, and an optional 30-min break period between the Perceptual Ability Test section and the Reading Comprehension Test Section. The 90-min Survey of the Natural Sciences section contains 100 questions, 40 of which come from Biology, while General Chemistry and Organic Chemistry evenly split the other 60. The PAT portion of the exam will only provide an hour for 90 questions. Test-takers will be provided 60 min for the Reading Comprehension Test, which contains 50 questions. The Quantitative Reasoning Test will offer 45 min to complete 50 questions, along with a basic four-function on-screen calculator to aid in completing the section. General breakdowns of what topics will be covered can be found in the ADA's DAT Guide and many studies aid companies, like Kaplan, have put together more in-depth breakdowns on how likely you are to see questions on certain subtopics (Kaplan, 2021).

Along with the Academic Average, which is what most people refer to as their DAT score, each subtopic will also be assigned its own score from 1–30. The test is standardized and graded on a bell curve. Each test-taker will receive a sub-score for each section, along with a Total Science score determined by the composite score of the biology and both chemistry sections. As of 2021, the national Academic Average for the DAT is a score of 19 (American Dental Association, 2021b). Many schools have lower limits for what they will accept in terms of sub-scores. Each school has different standards, so it is important to do research concerning the institutions you are interested in applying to. If you perform poorly on one or more subsections of the DAT and your attempt was later in the year, this may cause your application to remain incomplete until you are able to retake the exam 3 months later. This is just another reason why proper planning and time management is imperative.

Time management is an important skill to have for any person hoping to pursue a career in dentistry, regardless of their place in the process. In most cases, intensive and efficient studying is needed to score well on the DAT. Beyond that, some sections, such as PAT and Reading Comprehension, may pose a challenge to those who struggle to work quickly under time constraints. Due to the sections containing complex visual puzzles that generally require a decent amount of mental gymnastics to solve and long articles that might take a while to read and fully comprehend, timed practice is another necessary component when taking the DAT. Studying and practicing for such an intense, stamina-testing examination is critical to ensure an adequate performance on test day. The more you can put yourself in the testing mindset, the more comfortable you will feel when the day itself arrives.

So, how does one study effectively for a test that covers so much information? How do you practice effectively? We mentioned Kaplan and its test preparation resources earlier, but it is only one of the many third-party study materials made available to test-takers. Although the ADA provides old sample test material to aid students in preparation, it is imperative that students supplement their studies with helpful materials and study aids. Most use a combination of resources, while others find a program they like and stick with it. Many paid online options are available, such as DAT Bootcamp, DAT Destroyer, Crack the DAT, and more. Many big names in the study game, such as Kaplan, Khan Academy, and The Princeton Review, have put out their own DAT study materials. Some of these materials are available online, while others are physical copies that can be bought. They vary in price, from free to several hundreds or even thousands of dollars. Chad's Videos are a common paid online program that is not DAT-specific but has proven to be helpful. Many creators on YouTube, such as The Organic Chemistry Tutor, have also put out material specific to the DAT in addition to their other unrelated content. It isn't really a question of if there are study aids available, but more of a question of which ones you should use.

There are so many options available, and it can feel a bit overwhelming. How do you know what will work best for you? What's worth spending your time and money on? The truth is everyone's different! What works for you might not work for someone else and vice versa. One quick look at online community groups dedicated to the dental school application process will prove this point. Whether it's your DAT score or your GPA or when you get your interview invitation, everyone's journey will look different. Two people following the same study schedule using the same materials from the same program can end up with completely different results. However, as we saw in Chapter 5, two people who were accepted into the same dental school class will end up with totally different results as well. One will end up administering Botox and fillers and one will examine slides of biopsy samples all day. Therefore, comparing yourself to others in such a complex process will prove to be fruitless! Everyone will end up finding their own way that works for them. Some will get it right the first time, while others will take the DAT a couple of times before they achieve their desired scores. No patient will care how many times you had to take the DAT, and neither will you once you are a practicing dentist.

The AADSAS Application

The ADEA AADSAS usually opens at the beginning of June for applicants to apply to enter the incoming first-year classes of dental students across the United States for the following year. As of the 2021–2022 application cycle, the application fee will be $259 for the initial dental school and $112 for every additional school after that. Another update to the process will allow students to submit additional letters of recommendation along with their committee letter (American Dental Education Association: The Voice of Dental Education, 2021a). The application has four sections that must be completed: Personal Information, Academic History, Supporting Information, and Program Materials (American Dental Education Association: The Voice of Dental Education, 2021e).

The Personal Information section is where each applicant should store their most updated contact information, including the email address and street address at which they would like to receive all official correspondence. It is imperative to make a habit of checking your chosen email's junk or spam folder to avoid missing important alerts about your application status and possible interview invitations! This is also where the applicant will put their DENTPIN that will connect their DAT score(s) to their application.

The Academic History section is where the applicant will request official transcripts from all institutions where they have completed coursework and where they will enter test scores to be verified through the applicant's DENTPIN. The applicant must input all course information to be verified by the transcripts or must pay a fee to have the courses entered for them. This process of inputting the information must be carefully overseen to avoid errors. Any mistakes may cause the application process to be delayed.

The Supporting Information section is where the applicant will submit their personal statement and request letters of evaluation, also referred to as letters of recommendation. This section more than likely will require some thought and careful planning.

For the personal statement portion of the application, the prospective student should begin crafting their essay as soon as they feel as though they have their basic idea. The personal statement looks different for everybody (that's what makes it personal) and it needs to showcase the achievements, personality, and spirit of the applicant. Dental schools appreciate authenticity, so it is important to write a personal statement that highlights the best parts of you but also provides a realistic narrative about how you got to where you are and why you have ultimately chosen to pursue dentistry. Be yourself and share your story! This is where the admissions committee really gets a peak at the real you. While finding your voice may seem difficult and somewhat daunting at first, the right words will come to you when you get on the right track. Have peers and mentors read your personal statement and start getting used to receiving feedback on your work (you will do a lot of this in dental school). This may seem scary, but some of the best suggestions can come from someone else seeing what you have written with fresh eyes! Although feedback can be helpful, make sure to keep your personal statement personal and don't let anyone sway you on any of the parts you're sure about. If a new idea speaks to you, give it a chance! However, if someone tries to change the essence of what you're trying to communicate, make sure to stand behind what you have created and be proud of it (you will learn to do a lot of this in dental school as well). Let your personal statement become a mirror so that when the Dean of Admissions sees the words on the page, they see you.

As for your letters of evaluation, the AADSAS application allows an applicant to submit up to four letters and there are several different methods used to complete this step in the process. Figuring out which method your undergraduate institution is incredibly important. Some undergraduate institutions have committees, containing up to 15 individuals, that interview students and write committee letters or composite letters. Committee letters are written based on discussion following the applicant's interview with the committee. Generally, the committee leader will write a letter based on the comments of the group. On the other hand, composite letters often have several members write letters that will be combined, and the committee head will compose a cover letter for the combination of notes. Both types of letters count as three letters of evaluation. As noted earlier in the chapter, students can now submit additional letters of evaluation along with the committee and composite letters. The last type of letter accepted by the AADSAS application is referred to as the individual letter. These types of letters are usually sought out and procured by the student. Usually, applicants will ask professors, advisors, mentors, or dentists whom they have formed strong relationships within order to ensure that they will receive strong letters in their favor. If you are responsible for procuring your own letters, make sure to know the requirements, ask early, provide a reasonable timeline, and show your gratitude! Many schools have requirements or recommendations for whom individual letters should be written. Generally, schools are looking for two letters from two different science professors, one from an advisor, and one from a dentist, but it varies between institutions. Asking early is super important, especially with professors, since most upper-level science professors (especially the cool ones) have hundreds or even thousands of students hoping to get their own letter for whatever academic program or job they may be applying to. Get to the front of the line so a late letter submission doesn't hold up your application's completion. There is also no shame in asking your potential letter writers if they would be willing to write a strong recommendation in your favor. So many students make the mistake of assuming a professor advisor or dentist will write a strong letter for them just because they have shadowed them once or twice or shown their face at office hours before. Many letter writers have written about how they don't even know the student who asked for the letter, and some will submit letters that do not recommend the student for admission. This is not meant to scare you but to make you think long and hard about who you want to be your advocate in that admissions office. Make sure your letter writers know your due dates and expectations and let them know when you will be following up with them! Set reminders on your phone and send them reminders. Once they have completed your letter, show some appreciation for their time by treating them to a small gift or writing a simple thank you note! Their time is valuable and any person willing to write you a letter of recommendation is using a chunk of it to help you progress toward your goals. Remember this tip at interview time or really all the time! Some dental schools will ask for additional letters in their supplemental applications, so be prepared for that possibility (American Dental Education Association: The Voice of Dental Education, 2021f).

Program Materials is often the final completed section. This is where you will find supplemental information about the individual programs you are applying to and considering. Although you will spend most of your time perfecting the information in the other sections, do not overlook this one! Due to the cost of the application process, often nonrefundable deposits, and the amount of time and hard work that goes into applying to dental schools, it's also important to narrow down your top choices to a reasonable number. Of course, you want to give yourself the best chance at getting into school, but make sure to consider whether you will want to go to that school should you get accepted. Dental school is not a cheap investment, and it isn't like undergraduate institutions where you can transfer later if you aren't happy with your initial decision. A lot of thought should go into your decision, and you should consider several important factors, such as tuition and fees, location, curriculum, faculty-to-student ratio, class size, institutional values, along with many others. You know what is best for you and only you can decide which dental schools would be a good fit for you. Therefore, you must put the time in and do your research! This decision will affect the trajectory of your entire career and ultimately your life. Do not take it lightly.

Shadowing

Shadowing is an important aspect of every applicant's resume due to its ability to expose that person to dentistry and all the field has to offer. It is important to gain as much exposure to the profession before applying as possible, but it is equally important to be honest about the amount of time you have spent in a dental office. In the past, applicants with what some schools would consider too few shadowing hours have been asked how they even know dentistry is the right field for them. Other applicants with exorbitant shadowing hours have been asked to recall an entire dental procedure step-by-step. Knowing what dental schools are looking for when it comes to shadowing can help the applicant efficiently spend their time in dental offices learning, growing, and building relationships with dental healthcare professionals.

Asking a dentist you know personally, whether it be a family friend, a class speaker, or even your own dentist, if you can shadow them is a great place to start. Many dentists enjoy being shadowed! However, if they are unwilling to host you, they more than likely know someone who would be delighted to teach you more about dentistry. Before attending your first shadowing session, make sure to confirm appropriate attire, as well as the office rules and expectations.

It is important to shadow a general dentist to get a good idea of what dentistry is all about. After all, this is what you'll be doing in dental school, so you might as well learn now whether you will enjoy it enough to do it for at least 4 years (and more than likely, the rest of your life)! Once you've spent time learning the basics, you can branch out to specialties that interest you. Get started as early as you can and take advantage of different opportunities. Private practice is a huge part of the dental profession, but public health, corporate dentistry, academic dentistry, military dentistry, and so many more options are available if you only know how to look!

Generally, dental schools want to see you have spent an adequate amount of time observing dental procedures. Some schools require at least 100 hours of shadowing experience, but many recommend more. This is where time management and careful planning come into play again! With the COVID-19 pandemic, shadowing opportunities have become few and far between. An earlier start would have saved students several hours of watching crown prep videos on YouTube. Start early to take full advantage of the opportunities made available to you. This is going to be your life. Do your part to make sure you are investing your time, money, and effort wisely.

Community Service

Dentistry is a field of service. Every health care provider is serving their patients, and it is of utmost importance for dental schools to admit kind-hearted servant-leaders. Some may think of service as another shiny gold star on their resume, but dental schools see service-oriented individuals as future role models in the field of dentistry. While service opportunities can help further prove an applicant's dedication to the field, whether it be serving on dental mission trips or volunteering in public health clinics, dental schools love to see service of all kinds and, in a lot of cases, incorporate community service into their curricula!

Although service should be about the people you are serving and not just another checkbox on the road to dental school, the truth of the matter is that it is an important part of the application and an applicant with more community service hours is simply more attractive to admissions offices than those with totals on the lower side. Dental schools want well-rounded students who care about people just as much as they care about grades!

In terms of non-dental service, there are always a plethora of opportunities. Service is all about the heart, so find a cause you are passionate about and pour yourself into it! Whether you help at church, volunteer at the Special Olympics, or even just play with puppies at a shelter, there are so many great organizations with different needs that fit different people's personalities and schedules.

If you want to pour into your passion for dentistry, consider applying for a mission trip. Some trips can be taken for academic credit and are a great way to learn more about dentistry while serving those in need. Exercise caution when researching trips and make sure you will be performing a role you are qualified to do, such as shadowing or simply assisting. Rules can vary from country to country, and you obviously don't want to hurt your chances of gaining admission by participating in a trip that might not be completely legitimate. However, there are several reputable mission programs offered to undergraduate students that will allow you to gain firsthand exposure to dentistry in another country in a safe, exciting way. These experiences are priceless, and the knowledge and experience gained through them are invaluable. Mission trips are often offered during breaks by clubs run in conjunction with dental schools as well, so it's the perfect opportunity to test the waters before you end up being the one placing restorations and extracting teeth!

Unfortunately, the COVID-19 pandemic might end up changing the ways applicants can participate in dental service for good, so if you can't travel abroad, consider volunteering in free clinics here at home or asking a local dentist if they could use a volunteer or an intern. Although mission trips allow you to serve those in need all over the world, remember that there are plenty of people in need right in your backyard!

Whether you simply join a club that offers regular service opportunities in the local community or take a trip abroad to serve impoverished people groups, you can practice a life of service anywhere, anytime. Some schools look for a certain number of hours, like shadowing, but in all honesty, serving others needs to become an integral part of your lifestyle if you plan on becoming a successful health care provider. Taking care of people is what you will do for a living and serving your patients will become your life's purpose!

Research

Academic research is another great opportunity to learn more about the dental field (or any scientific field that interests you really) in a way that will impress admissions committees across the United States. Being a published author is a thrilling achievement for any person, but to be able to participate in published research before you have even obtained your first doctorate is not something you should take for granted. University professors are often teaching to fund their research trials, so reach out to the professor of your favorite science class and see if they have any interest in taking on an undergraduate assistant. The experience gained from conducting research will be attractive to dental schools but will also provide you the satisfaction of knowing you have personally contributed to the progression of modern science.

Manual Dexterity

Admissions committees are also interested in seeing if applicants can walk the walk, not just talk the talk. Developing hand skills is an extremely vital part of dental education. Working to develop these hand skills is built into the dental curriculum, so having incredible hand skills right off the bat is not a prerequisite for admission. However, a natural knack for fine motor movements can pique the interest of admissions committees. Whether you play an instrument, practice calligraphy, crochet, knit, or even just play a lot of video games, proof that you are working on fine-tuning your hand–eye coordination (intentionally or not) before admission is attractive to dental institutions (American Dental Education Association: The Voice of Dental Education, 2021h).

Interviews and the Waiting Game

If you have finally completed your application and ensured that every single step has been taken care of, all you can really do now is... Wait. If any of the schools you apply to happen to pass you through to interviews, you will receive an interview invitation. Some schools call, some email (keep checking that spam folder!), and some send snail mail. Keep your eyes peeled for any official correspondence and be prompt in responding! Interview slots fill up quickly and there is always someone waiting in line to take that spot, so you must act fast to ensure you get your chance to interview. Every school is different, and every interview process varies from institution to institution. Read about the specific school's interview process on forums or online groups. Better yet, if you know someone who goes to the school in real life, ask for tips or advice. The more familiar you are with the flow of things, the more comfortable you will be on the big day. Obviously, you want to be prepared, but too much practice can leave you sounding over-rehearsed. You can memorize and recite answers to sample interview questions until you are blue in the face, but once the adrenaline starts pumping, you'll forget everything you had written in your four-page outline of your extensive answer to the question, "Why dentistry?" The best thing you can do for yourself is to get a professional outfit that you feel great in, take time to appreciate the chance you have been given, and just be yourself. If you have followed the advice in these pages up until now, the person the admissions committee chose to meet with is *you*. You made it this far and now all you must do is show up, smile, and remind them why they gave you the interview in the first place.

After the interview is over, it's back to waiting ... Again. The days, weeks, or months between interview day and decision day will seem like forever. Some will be lucky and get good news on day one, while others will wait for months and months, scouring the Student Doctor Network for updates from other newly accepted students. There is really nothing that can ease the mind of an anxious applicant waiting by the computer. However, do your best to relax. You have done all that you can do, and the waiting will eventually end. Just try to enjoy your last few months of life before dental school (or life before you begin the process all over again). The road to dental school is long, but for those who gain acceptance, it finally ends and officially marks the beginning of a brand-new journey: the road to becoming a dentist!

References

American Dental Association (2021a). Dental admission test. Retrieved from https://www.ada.org/en/education-careers/dental-admission-test

American Dental Association (2021b). Dental admission test: Frequently asked questions about scoring. Retrieved from https://www.ada.org/~/media/ADA/Education%20and%20Careers/Files/dat_scoring_faq.pdf?la=en

American Dental Association (2021c). Take the DAT at a prometric test center. Retrieved from https://www.ada.org/en/education-careers/dental-admission-test/take-the-dat-at-a-prometric-test-center

American Dental Education Association: The Voice of Dental Education (2021a). ADEA AADSAS application updates. Retrieved from https://www.adea.org/GoDental/ADEAAADSASApplicationUpdates/

American Dental Education Association: The Voice of Dental Education (2021b). ADEA AADSAS participating dental schools required and recommended courses. Retrieved from https://www.adea.org/uploadedFiles/GoDental/Prehealth_Advisors/Getting_into_Dental_School/ADEAAADSASRequiredandRecommendedCourses_FINAL002).pdf

American Dental Education Association: The Voice of Dental Education (2021c). Application prep. Retrieved from https://www.adea.org/GoDental/Application_Prep.aspx

American Dental Education Association: The Voice of Dental Education (2021d). College major. Retrieved from https://www.adea.org/GoDental/Application_Prep/Preparing_for_Dental_School/College_major.aspx

American Dental Education Association: The Voice of Dental Education (2021e). Dental school applicant quick guide. Retrieved from https://www.adea.org/GoDental/The_application_to_dental_school__ADEA_AADSAS.aspx

American Dental Education Association: The Voice of Dental Education (2021f). Letters of evaluation. Retrieved from https://www.adea.org/GoDental/Application_Prep/The_Admissions_Process/Letters_of_evaluation.aspx

American Dental Education Association: The Voice of Dental Education (2021g). Preparing for dental school. Retrieved from https://www.adea.org/GoDental/Application_Prep/Preparing_for_dental_school.aspx

American Dental Education Association: The Voice of Dental Education (2021h). The importance of manual dexterity. Retrieved from https://www.adea.org/GoDental/Application_Prep/Preparing_for_Dental_School/The_Importance_of_Manual_Dexterity.aspx

Kaplan. (2021). DAT study tips & resources. https://www.kaptest.com/study/dat/

CHAPTER 7

Dental Care in the United States

Anna Foster Crowe

The Status of Dental Care in the United States

As soon as you begin serving patients in dental school, you are beginning your career as a dental clinician! While this is exciting, the occupation comes with a lot of responsibilities. Oral health care is incredibly important, and the oral cavity is often considered the window to the rest of the body. Therefore, an emphasis on maintaining oral health is of paramount importance. However, much like other fields of health care in the United States, there is no guarantee that every U.S. resident will receive dental care.

Although there have been drastic improvements in the population's general oral health in the past several years, there are still disparities in this country concerning who is able to receive care. Public dental clinics are even harder to come by than medical clinics and patients often struggle to procure quality care if they do not have dental insurance. Resources that many communities in the United States are afforded are glaringly absent from others, such as a fluoridated community water source or free dental health programs provided for elementary-age children. Although Medicare has not covered dental health services in the past, the topic is up for debate as new legislation is currently being presented to change that. This is controversial among providers and laypeople alike, but the inclusion of dental coverage in Medicare plans would help elderly individuals, who are disproportionately underserved, gain access to quality dental care even after retirement.

Socioeconomic status is another consideration when looking at the lack of dental care in the population. Medicaid plans are not required to include dental coverage and currently, 13 states require no coverage or only emergency coverage to be provided. Caries, or tooth decay, are rampant in nearly half of low-income individuals and have been exhibited in Black individuals at disproportionate rates. In adults and children, obvious differences in oral health status can be observed in Black and Hispanic individuals when compared with White individuals. Older Black and Hispanic individuals, as well as smokers, are also more likely to suffer from gum disease. Oral cancer is also more likely to be fatal in Black men than in White men (Centers for Disease Control and Prevention, 2021).

Many improvements can still be made to the field of oral health care, but if the progress made in the past 50 years is any indication of the current trajectory, the future of dentistry has an optimistic air surrounding it. The best thing dental clinicians can do to ensure a better future for the field is to champion public dental health programs and work hard every day to personally contribute to more equitable access to dental care for all.

Recent Changes in Dental Health Care

In addition to the recent vast improvements to the overall accessibility of dentistry, even though there is undoubtedly still work to do, technology continues to progress, which in turn is allowing dentistry to become faster, more efficient, and more cost-effective for patients and providers alike. Digital dentistry has unlocked so many possibilities and is allowing clinicians to provide more effective care to their patient populations.

The regular usage of CAD/CAM digital scanners and three-dimensional printers will soon render outdated traditional techniques obsolete and tedious procedures that used to take weeks will now take only a few hours. There are even several different ways that technology assists providers in more serious procedures! Fluorescence imaging and dental cone beam computer tomography images can assist providers in surgeries and even diagnoses of oral cancer (Colgate-Palmolive Company, 2021). These invaluable tools will further raise the standard of patient safety in oral health care. Other technologies are currently being implemented into the field of dentistry in several ways such as artificial intelligence, augmented and virtual reality, telehealth, the use of stem cells for regenerative purposes, and even genome editing (The Medical Futurist, 2020)! Whether it's leaders in oral hygiene providing apps that help people see what areas they need to focus on when brushing or researchers using stem cells to replace dental pulp in a tooth, so many great things are in development that will more than likely come to fruition within the career-span of prospective students currently applying to dental school. Much like the introduction of radiographs and electronic records, the introduction of these new technological advancements will most certainly change the field forever.

There have been many positive developments in the field recently, but not all changes have had a beneficial impact on dentistry. The COVID-19 pandemic, which is on track to become the deadliest event in U.S. history by the end of 2021, has already changed dentistry so much in its short life. There has not been such a drastic change in personal protective equipment protocols within the scope of dentistry since the beginning of the AIDS epidemic (*The New York Times*, 1987). Not only have personal protection protocols drastically changed, but many clinicians are also having to make several changes to the way they practice to ensure the health and safety of themselves, their staff, and their patients. Despite early reports that dental professionals were at a higher risk of contracting COVID-19 due to the mechanism of spread and the abundance of aerosols produced in procedures, the American Dental Association (ADA) stated that the infection rate of dentists was only 2.6% at the end of 2020. The ADA also noted that the risk for dental professionals was much less than originally reported (The American Dental Association News, 2021). The most important thing for providers is to remain vigilant and up to date on all forthcoming research.

Corporate Dentistry

Dental service organizations, also known as dental support organizations (DSOs), are corporate organizations that partner with practices to provide dental services under a single corporation's name (Dentistry iQ, 2016). Some of these organizations, like Heartland Dental, expanded to become the large networks they are today from smaller hubs, while others market a specific brand and partner with individual practice locations, like Aspen Dental. Another well-known DSO, Affordable Dentures, provides specialized care in a specific area of dentistry under its recognizable brand.

Many providers express their disdain for DSOs because of the numbers-driven business model that so many follow. A good portion of clinicians feel as though corporate organizations prey on young dentists hoping to be paid well to start paying off loans and overwork them to meet quotas without really emphasizing the quality of the work. While some DSOs may follow this methodology, it is impossible to speak for every large corporation and their personal intentions. Dental service organizations are not going anywhere either due to changes trending in favor of larger businesses in terms of insurance reimbursements. Dr. Kevin Cain expects dentistry to follow the same shift as pharmacy did, with dentists becoming more often providers for a larger brand than their own boss in private practice. Due to the "business first" mode of operation fueling so many DSOs, they can efficiently run their practices well with optimized overhead costs. To compete and obtain similar levels of success and profitability, Dr. Cain believes private practitioners must learn to play the game the DSOs are playing to survive (The American Dental Association News, 2021). Despite Dr. Cain's claims, many recently graduated clinicians are still finding plenty of success in private practice, whether as owners or associates. However, with the ever-growing cost of becoming a dentist, it is surely becoming increasingly more difficult for younger dentists to ignore the occupational and financial security that working for a DSO can provide.

Choices

Because of the several types of practices, residency programs, and auxiliary positions, it is obvious that dentistry is an expansive and growing field full of endless opportunities. As we discussed in earlier chapters, a couple of new specialties were recently recognized, and the field continues to grow every year. Whether you are just applying or simply curious as to what dentistry could possibly offer you, the extremely varied options available to someone hoping to pursue a career in dentistry are evident. After reading about all the requirements and steps, maybe you're realizing the path to dentistry is more involved than you are prepared for now. On the other hand, maybe this information inspired you to chase your dream of becoming an orthodontist or an oral maxillofacial surgeon. A passion for oral health care does not lead everyone down the same path and luckily, we can choose the occupation that best fits our personal skillset. Whether you become a lab technician, an assistant, a hygienist, or a dentist, every piece of the puzzle matters and plays a critical role in the maintenance of the oral health of the general population in the United States. If making people smile is your top priority, you are on the right track!

Future

One aspect that will influence the practice of dentistry across the board will be whether dental services will be at long last be included as a reimbursable expenditure in the realm of Medicare and Medicaid to provide coverage for dental services to all especially those citizens who have been traditionally underserve and/or lack health insurance for whatever reason. To date, dental and optical clinical services have not been included as part of the health coverage provided under the health social safety nets provided by the federal government. Unfortunately, to expand this universal health policy for all citizens is not supported by the ADA. The reasons for their lack of support are based on concerns that if enacted the rate of reimbursement to dental practitioners would not accurately reflect their time and effort to deliver dental procedures, in addition to provide for full cost recovery to deliver those dental services. Lost in this debate is the basic premise—oral health is the key component to basic overall health status for every man, woman, and child; therefore, to ignore or disallow opportunities to expand dental services to populations that are most in need is disingenuous to these citizens as well as poor clinical practice. Hopefully, the legislation providing for expanded health care coverage to include dental services will be enacted sooner rather than later. Time will tell.

References

Centers for Disease Control and Prevention (2021). Disparities in oral health. Retrieved from https://www.cdc.gov/oralhealth/oral_health_disparities/index.htm

Colgate-Palmolive Company (2021). The changing world of digital dentistry. Retrieved from https://www.colgate.com/en-us/oral-health/dental-visits/the-changing-world-of-digital-dentistry

Dentistry iQ (2016). Corporate dentistry defined. Retrieved from https://www.dentistryiq.com/practice-management/industry/article/16366546/corporate-dentistrydefined

The American Dental Association News (2021). ADA tells White House: No 'grave danger' of being exposed to COVID-19 in dental settings. Retrieved from https://www.ada.org/en/publications/ada-news/2021-archive/june/ada-tells-white-house-no-grave-danger-of-being-exposed-to-covid-19-in-dental-settings#:~:text=O'Loughlin%2C%20D.M.D.%2C%20noted,availability%20of%20COVID%2D19%20vaccines

The Medical Futurist (2020). Technologies that will shape the future of dentistry. Retrieved from https://medicalfuturist.com/the-amazing-future-of-dentistry-and-oral-health/

The New York Times (1987). AIDS precautions taken by dentists. Retrieved from https://www.nytimes.com/1987/06/06/nyregion/aids-precautions-taken-by-dentists.html

Contributor Biography

Anna Foster-Crowe

Ms. Foster-Crowe is a graduate of the Dental College of Georgia, Augusta, GA. She received her BS degree in biological sciences from Clemson University in 2019. She is a practicing dentist in Seneca, SC.